Nursing Informatics

Nursing Informatics
Connecting Technology and Patient Care

First Edition

By Priscilla O. Okunji

Howard University

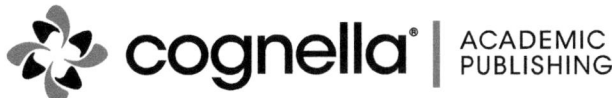

Bassim Hamadeh, CEO and Publisher
Carrie Montoya, Manager, Revisions and Author Care
Amy Smith, Project Editor
Christian Berk, Associate Production Editor
Emely Villavicencio, Senior Graphic Designer
Sara Schennum, Licensing Associate
Natalie Piccotti, Senior Marketing Manager
Kassie Graves, Vice President of Editorial
Jamie Giganti, Director of Academic Publishing

Copyright © 2019 by Cognella, Inc. All rights reserved. No part of this publication may be reprinted, reproduced, transmitted, or utilized in any form or by any electronic, mechanical, or other means, now known or hereafter invented, including photocopying, microfilming, and recording, or in any information retrieval system without the written permission of Cognella, Inc. For inquiries regarding permissions, translations, foreign rights, audio rights, and any other forms of reproduction, please contact the Cognella Licensing Department at rights@cognella.com.

Trademark Notice: Product or corporate names may be trademarks or registered trademarks, and are used only for identification and explanation without intent to infringe.

Cover image copyright © 2017 iStockphoto LP/Elenabs.

Printed in the United States of America.

ISBN: 978-1-62661-624-0 (pbk) / 978-1-62661-625-7 (br)

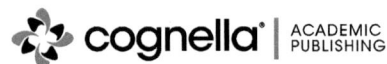

Brief Contents

Preface   vii

Unit I

1 Informatics in Today's Healthcare   3
2 Computer, Operating System and Software   13
3 Computer Networks, Applications, Concerns, and Security Measures   25

Unit II

4 An Overview of Nursing Informatics   37
5 External Drivers of Informatics Technology   49
6 Nurse Executives and the Use of Informatics in Documentation and Other Administrative Activities   53

Unit III

7 Systems Interoperability and Levels of Standardization   63
8 Data Mining and Knowledge Discovery   77
9 Data and Evidence-Based Research in Nursing   83

Unit IV

10 E-Health: Disease Prevention and Management   121
11 Health Information Systems and Patient Safety   133
12 Health Information Confidentiality, Security, and Integrity   167

Unit V

13 Digital Library and Mobile Computing   183
14 E-Learning, Teaching, and Author's Related Projects   189
15 Faculty Development via Author's Selected Scholarly E-Learning Articles   205

Preface

JUST AS NURSE educators are continuously challenged to stay current in today's complex healthcare, the environment continues to rapidly expand in the field of nursing informatics. An excerpt from the 2016 National Nursing Informatics Deep Dive conference very well highlighted the urgency as follows:

> Nurse educators' expectation ranges from electronic health records, social media, consumer informatics, mobile-health, smart phones, and other applications to prepare students for a data, information, and technology intensive healthcare environment. In addition, there is high expectations from "digital natives" or students who have grown up in the information age and already possess advanced computer skills. [Information technology is an enabling tool that links] data, information, knowledge and wisdom and facilitates problem solving and decision making. However, incorporating information technology in ways that educate students on these important concepts remains a challenge for many educators and this is the real focus of writing this Nursing Informatics in higher education. The growing impact of information technology on the delivery of care, professional nursing organizations have resulted in the establishment of standards for nursing informatics to assist faculty [to] integrate the skills into program curriculums. These standards include The AACN Essentials of Baccalaureate Education for Professional Nursing Practice Information Management and Application of Patient Care Technology, The TIGER Informatics Competencies for Every Practicing Nurse and The QSEN Knowledge, Skills and Attitudes for Informatics. (National Nursing Informatics Deep Dive Program, 2016)

Hence, the aforementioned rationale has prompted the author into writing her original book that should enable students understand more of the use of nursing informatics in higher education. In addition to the introduction of nursing informatics, the use of computers in healthcare, and others, this text will align these standards with suggested learning methods, tools, and learning resources to teach students. Faculty development in online teaching and learning program creation was included as well. The text should not be limited to only undergraduate students, as graduate students need informatics in their curriculum. The text could be used in graduate and certificate programs as nursing informatics competency is now expected to be integrated across the nursing curriculum in all higher institutions that offer nursing programs (Table 0.1).

As an instructor, the author did spearhead the planning, development and implementation of the online RN-BSN program and the traditional nursing informatics courses in

TABLE 0.1 Competency Matrix for Nursing Informatics

Levels	AACN BSN Essentials	TIGER Competency	QSEN Undergraduate KSA's	AACN Essential Masters	QSEN Graduate KSA's	AACN Essential DNP
Undergraduate	✓	✓	✓			
Masters	✓	✓	✓	✓	✓	
DNP	✓	✓	✓	✓	✓	✓

Peri (2018)

2010 and 2011, respectively. In addition, the author coordinated the online program from 2011–2016 and single handedly taught the traditional undergraduate informatics course students at Howard University's College of Nursing and Allied Health Sciences until the 2016 fall semester. The first book the author used, in 2010, in informatics and technology was an existing book and the content was not what she expected informatics should be in nursing, as the department was revamping the curriculum according to AACN standards. After the author's second year of teaching and evaluation of the text (2011–2012), she selected a second text because it was closer to what she wanted the students to learn and practice in nursing informatics. However, to make the students understand that the essence of nursing informatics is not to become an information technologist, rather that it's the use of technology to manage information, she began to customize the course activities in a way that the students would relate to the course as what nurses do daily as knowledge workers. Currently, nursing schools are incorporating informatics into their nursing curriculum, and the author has become a resource to the clinical course coordinators in the incorporation of nursing informatics in the undergraduate curriculum because of the following believe:

- Nursing informatics is composed of required nursing standards/competencies, as in AACN Essentials of Baccalaureate Education for Professional Nursing Practice, Information Management and Application of Patient Care Technology, the TIGER Informatics Competencies for Every Practicing Nurse, and the QSEN Knowledge, Skills and Attitudes for Informatics (KSA)
- An electronic EHR simulation is needed in the nursing clinical courses prior to actual clinicals in healthcare institutions
- NCLEX questions on patient confidentiality, security, privacy (HIPAA), analytics, and safety are informatics related because informatics primary outcomes in patients' admission are shorter LOS, more discharges/admissions, and increased patients' satisfaction—hence more money for the healthcare institution
- Other added values in this text include health literacy, numeracy, authors research and publications to assist faculty development in the creation of online programs

- In addition, the author was able to customize the courses through the integration of an assessment tool and its responses that would enable understanding of the students' knowledge about informatics and learning methods preferences prior to each class, as depicted in the links below:
  1. Google form page: https://docs.google.com/forms/d/1j-aVTpF6P3H4E-OigkByfw7i4dunVYnl5mv5f4viH0Q/viewform?edit_requested=true
  2. Survey Responses: https://docs.google.com/forms/d/1j-aVTpF6P3H4E-OigkByfw7i4dunVYnl5mv5f4viH0Q/viewanalytics?pli=1

- Video making as a practical activity for students in any course is a plus (students enjoy the group activities). The 2012 class assignment was one of the videos for an award-winning "Teaching with Technology" (http://www.cetla.howard.edu/featured_teacher/archive/okunji.html)
  - The author was glad to find some of the students' owned public websites, for the directed innovative group projects associated with the Informatics course. The students enjoyed making the videos as depicted in the below links:
    1. http://youtu.be/E8UEo0-hY88
    2. https://youtube.com/watch?v=QBJJZzc84DI
    3. http://youtu.be/O_2IL1uDIOY
    4. https://youtu.be/uYWxQkKZAXw
    5. https://youtu.be/LuSGPXIiT68

Other inclusions are samples of data analytics and teaching tools and methods:

- Detailed data acquisition inclusion as it relates to what nurses do every day as knowledge workers and as is evidenced by online students' data acquisition, analysis, and presentation at conferences from 2014–2018.
- Data analysis using different statistical packages as they relate to research for both undergraduate and graduate students.
- Students' experience and case study scenarios, which are comprehensive or detailed, for student assignments at the end of the chapter (used with students' informed consent).
- A lab that was incorporated as a hybrid, alternating with classes for traditional students, as students' interaction and hands on are the most important variables in hybrid and online classes.
- An EHR simulation tool that was introduced using SimChart for competencies and for students who want to be more hands on in the computer lab.

References

University of Minnesota. (2016). National Nursing Informatics Deep Dive Program. Retrieved from https://www.nursing.umn.edu/outreach/professional-development/national-nursing-informatics-deep-dive-program

Peri, J. (2018). Infusing digital health technology across the curriculum (presentation). National Nursing Informatics Conference; Tampa, Florida.

UNIT I

CHAPTER 1

Informatics in Today's Healthcare

CHAPTER HIGHLIGHTS

This chapter discusses the following:

- How changing needs have impacted healthcare costs, leading to an increased need for healthcare-related technology
- How the increased use of technology requires healthcare professionals to have a high level of proficiency in working with technology for satisfactory patients' care.
- How the government, patients, and healthcare providers have been the forces driving a move toward a greater use of informatics
- How the effects of informatics on healthcare would force nurses to be computer fluent and information literate to face the challenges of today's healthcare
- A students' perspective on "What Informatics Is and What It Is Not" and "Nursing Informatics and Technology"

WHEN SOCIETY CHANGES, SO DOES HEALTHCARE: THE CALL FOR HEALTHCARE INFORMATICS

THE CHANGING SOCIETAL needs have led to an increase in healthcare costs and health provider shortages, which has led the administrators to call for new designs in healthcare delivery. Information technology (IT) and skills training are being included in the current nursing education curriculum. In other words, everyday nursing students are being trained to use computer technology to meet the expectations of the nursing profession. This contemporary form of nursing practice in hospital units entails the use of computers that meet specific hardware criteria and PC software such as word processing, spreadsheets and databases, with the common goal of improving patient safety and satisfaction while making the workflow for nurses more efficient.

The proliferation of computers has highlighted the importance of the discussion of nurses' expectations as nursing informatics has become critical in today's nursing practice, especially in education. This is needed to prepare future nurses for current and paperless health institutions. It is rare to peruse any recent scholarly paper without noticing a nursing informatics component, as these skills are critically needed for positive outcomes of the patients. Hence, the expectation is that nurses should be able to work with various types of information and communication technologies to be relevant in today's healthcare environment.

> The delivery of timely clinical data and relevant clinical evidence to nurses is crucial in any re-design of healthcare processes. Nursing provides a critical link in the co-ordination of patient care within healthcare organizations. Registered nurses (RNs) are the largest number of direct healthcare providers in the United States[;] as of March 2000[,] an estimated 2,201,813 RNs were employed in nursing within the United States. Information systems have the ability to change raw data into information that can enhance the nursing process. (Courtney, Demiris, & Alexander, 2005)

This change can be seen with the transformation of displaying data graphically over time. Information management encompasses computer technology and people; the underpinning of Informatics is to produce qualified nursing information technology professionals who utilize information in problem solving, innovation, communication, and teamwork. Among the approaches for mastering this act are understanding computer software, information management, the basic features and operating functions of computers and their language, algorithms, the importance of user groups, and software copyright and piracy law. With introduction of electronic health records (EHR), the knowledge and efficient use of system and application software and features will greatly impact nurses' productivity whether the nurse is beginning, well experienced, or is a nurse informatics specialist.

The focus of the next section is to give the overview of some of the forces driving a move toward a greater use of informatics, distinguish between informatics, and analyze the effects of informatics on healthcare and the need for nurses to be computer fluent and information literate to face the challenges of today's healthcare.

FORCES BEHIND THE MOVE TOWARD INFORMATICS

Some of the forces behind the movement toward a greater use of informatics include national forces, nursing forces, patient safety, and cost.

National Forces

The federal efforts behind a move to electronic health records (EHR) also include standardization of data. The Institute of Medicine (IOM), an independent body that acts as an adviser to the U.S. government completed several reports aimed at improving healthcare, all of which foresee a large role for IT. In 2004, President Bush called for the adoption of interoperable EHR's for most Americans by 2014. He established the position of national coordinator for Health Information Technology. The 2008–2012 strategic plan was released to address "the federal activities necessary to achieve the nationwide implementation of this technology infrastructure throughout both the public and private sectors." The strategic plan formulated two goals that affect nurses and healthcare:

a. Patient-focused healthcare: Provide higher quality, cost-efficient care using electronic information exchange among healthcare providers, patients, and their designees. The strategies for achieving these goals are as follows:
   - To facilitate electronic exchange of the patient's health information while protecting privacy and security of the information
   - To make the information exchange interoperable so that it is available when and where needed
   - To promote nationwide adoption of EHRs and personal health records
   - To establish collaborative governance to guide the health information technology infrastructure
b. Population health: Allow for access and "use of electronic health information to support public health, biomedical research, quality improvement, and emergency preparedness." The strategies are as follows:
   - To provide for information access and use of population while protecting privacy and security of the information
   - To make the information exchange interoperable to support population-oriented uses
   - To promote nationwide adoption of technologies and technical functions that will improve population and individual health
   - To establish collaborative governance to support the information use of population health

It is clearly seen from these goals that paper format can no longer support the amount of information needed.

Nursing Forces

Nursing has also recognized the need for information and the value of data and insisted that the American Nurses Association (ANA) and the National League for Nurses (NLN) should make nursing information a priority. In 1993, the National Center for Nursing Research released the report "Nursing Informatics: Enhancing Patient Care," with the following six program goals for nursing informatics research:

- Establish nursing language (useful in computerized documentation)
- Develop methods to build clinical information databases
- Determine how nurses give patient care
- Develop and test patient care decision support systems
- Develop workstations that provide nurses with the needed information
- Develop appropriate methods to evaluate nursing information systems
- The Technology Informatics Guiding Educational Reform (TIGER) objective is to empower nurses and make informatics a primary focus of the 21st century. Poorly organized documentation and implementation systems hinder the process of finding and using the information one needs to provide high-quality care.

Patient Safety and Cost

Patient safety and the cost of care is a primary concern and is one of the main objectives driving informatics to a new level. With the American Recovery and Reinvestment Act signed into law, the American Academy of Nurses called on former President Obama's administration, Congress, technology manufacturers and purchasers to work with nurses and other healthcare providers to ensure that technologies are developed and deployed in a way that will allow healthcare providers more time with their patients, which resulted in increased safety, improved clinical outcomes and decreased cost. Both ANA and AACN have identified the need for both computer and information literacy skills as necessary for evidence-based practice. The American Nurses Association recognized nursing informatics as a subspecialty of nursing in 1992. Management of information pertaining to nursing is the primary objective in nursing informatics.

THE BENEFITS OF INFORMATICS IN HEALTHCARE

Each healthcare discipline will benefit from its investment in informatics because it will enhance the practice and development of nursing. It will improve documentation when properly implemented, which will ultimately reduce the amount of time spent in documentation. Nurses spend more time in documenting patient care and entering vital signs in nursing notes and flow sheets, which sometimes can create errors. Informatics makes clinical documentation of data easy, which will entail entering data once, and then it can be retrieved and presented in many different forms to meet the needs of the user. The ability to use patient data for both quality control and research will be greatly improved when documentation is complete and electronic.

Some of the benefits/effects of informatics on healthcare is that previously buried data, which is inaccessible, can now be easily retrieved and accessed. Informatics is not only collecting data, but making the data useful. When data are captured electronically in a structured manner, it can be retrieved and used in different ways. Informatics has made it possible for healthcare providers to communicate with each order, which will improve patient care and a better work environment. Information technology (IT) has made storage and retrieval of healthcare records easier. Computerized administrative tasks such as staffing and scheduling have become easier, which in turn saves money and time.

Student Experience: What Informatics Is and What It Is Not

Whittney M. Russell. RN, BSN

Each day, the patient encounters nursing and other healthcare support staff as the data grows and more documentation is added to the patient profile for future reference.

The data collected is entered primarily through computer systems that systematically process through the computer, software, and peripheral devices that are critical functional components of the computer. However, each computer system needs an operating system to function appropriately as required. Operating system, as defined by Merriam-Webster, is the collection of software that directs a computer's operations, controlling and scheduling the execution of other programs, and managing storage, input/output, and communication resources. These parts of the systems all operate together in performing function and output. I like to think of the hospital in the same context, as a multidisciplinary team dedicated to working together to provide care for the patients, in delivering quality care and promoting improved patient outcomes (webopedia, 2015).

This task has been made easier through the use of information technology. Not only has information technology made it easier to record data, but it has also made it easier for healthcare providers to retrieve information on previous treatments, care plans, testing, admissions information, laboratory results, and all other encounters that patients have had in the system, and have given staff an alternative for placing records from other facilities through scanning and downloading. In care for a complex patient or patient who has been in a healthcare system for an extended period of time, the hard-drives are crucial in maintaining information to assess the patient and establish goals effectively.

When I began working in an acute care hospital, I started out on a Medical Surgical unit that ran using paper charting and cardexes. Every time the patient was admitted, a new chart and cardex was started. Brand new demographic information, notes, labs, test results and radiography documents were recorded. Assessment data had to be conducted over and over with no account for what the patient's baseline health had been during the previous admission unless they were "frequent flyers." That was the term we used for patients whose health baseline and care plan were well known amongst staff, so we already knew what to expect or remembered information from a previous admission.

Care for the patient would slow dramatically throughout the day and care would often be delayed because there was only one source to collect and enter data concerning the patient's health. Everything, including orders would have to be reviewed in one chart and cardex. This meant that we all were waiting around to chart and get orders because we had to take turns with the chart and as always physicians were always allowed.

When the patient left the unit, so did that chart and the waiting game continued; we would often have to document later at the end of the shift, which caused staff to remain at work sometimes hours after the shift had ended, often not recording critical information because it was forgotten; nurses were mentally and physically drained and had to get home to their families or no longer spend time in charting. Sometimes critical information was not handed off to the on-coming shift because the chart was not there as a reference. Even worse, nurses would miss orders after not having access to the chart all day, leaving excess work on the next shift, causing tension between colleagues on the unit. After the patient had been discharged, all that vital information was bound and picked up by an individual from the records office and mostly never seen again. Information that could be used for a future admission, and to evaluate the outcome of care planning and its effectiveness, was locked away and the process would begin again on the next admission. It was completely inefficient in so many ways.

In 2004, President Bush incorporated the use of electronic health records (EHR) by the year 2014. Research has been conducted on the EMR vs. the paper medical record. In a study conducted in a Northeastern urban hospital between May and July of 2004, the records of 5 patients were reviewed that showed a complete documentation of inpatient and outpatient care. Data were recorded and compared with the data retrieved from the EMR of each patient. It was observed that not all the interfaces communicated with one another. The authors' results showed that electronic records were also problematic because of the difficulties in finding comparable data. This was due to each department style of documentation tool being used, not focus documentation and was due to the terms used in describing the information in the chart differing between departments in the hospital. It was found that the EMR did not function or give enough areas for comprehensive documentation as though it were written, and therefore, a lot of data had been missed when transferring written documentation to the programming. However, the study did find that that the EMR did help bridge the gap between obtaining information between inpatient and outpatient care (Smith, 2006).

In other research, it was found in the parallel use of electronic and paper charts; inconsistencies were present with the use of both forms of charting. The conclusion was that the implementation of electronic record systems intended to operate in parallel with paper-based systems, whose focus should be on securing the validity of all versions of the record. This research is important because, although most systems have now converted, paper is still used in most settings to evaluate particulars and then that data is imported into the EMR (Mikkelsen, 2001).

In regards to the nursing practice, specialized fields in informatics have developed with the purpose for bridging the gap between the use of paper records and future use of the computer and applications as tools in the workplace. The skill set of the Nurse Informatics specialist is to help transition healthcare informatics to the Nursing clinician and other subspecialties. However, the overall competency in usage of the informatics systems is based on those individuals' computer literacy and computer fluency. The nurse clinician and those in other fields must be able to find pertinent information, be able to evaluate it, and use it effectively in order to impact patient care in a positive way. The misuse of information technology can lead to undesirable patient outcomes and mismanagement of resources during the patients care in the inpatient and outpatient settings (Sewell & Thede, 2013).

During the transition from paper to electronic charting at my hospital, there was definitely a learning disparity amongst those individuals who had been practicing with paper charts over a long career vs. their peers who were younger and more accustomed to using computer systems. For those individuals, the hospital put in place extra classes and made people available as champions in certain areas who could be used as a reference for staff not so comfortable with the transition. Even still, there was worry amongst those individuals that they would not be able to give their patients the same quality of care they once did. In the end, most individuals did come around and began to work smoothly with the operating system.

The computer, however, is still only a tool to be used by the healthcare professional. The focus has always been and should continue to be the patient, positive outcomes, and quality care. There is research being conducted now as to why healthcare professionals are not implementing the rapid response systems and factors leading to this. Though the research continues, I would argue that computer systems and time spent away from patients is a factor. So often nurses are compelled to step away from the bedside to complete the charting that is required by the computer systems in order to avoid a multitude of red flag alerts on the screen at the end of the day. I feel like this leaves patients vulnerable, because the nurse is no longer as attentive as once before (Marshall, 2011).

There were a couple of occasions where I remember getting a report and it consisted of the off-going nurse telling me how the patient slept through the night and the vitals and labs were stable, and then I walk in and it is completely different from what had been reported. I feel it is because vitals are taken by the technician most of the time, and labs and other findings are located on the EMR. I found that after an initial assessment, some practitioners would end up nursing the computers and charting and forget to check the patient. In nursing school, I was always reminded to check the patient because as anyone who has worked on telemetry unit can tell you, the actual assessment of a patient can lead to much different findings that what data has been collected and the browsing of the EMR. The computer and its use for information management are undeniably important. However, the computer should be used as a tool and the patient should remain the focus.

Student Experience: Nursing Informatics and Technology

Denise Cabell, RN, BSN

Nursing informatics has created a job title for some nurses. It is a field that is very demanding and requires extensive clinical experience. Sixty-six percent of most nursing informacists have on average a total of 11-16 years of clinical experience and more than half have graduate degrees. This suggests that many nursing informacists went back to school for an advanced degree. A number of issues pose problems for nursing informacists in the field. Lack of integration in computer systems and software, inadequate financial resources, lack of administrative support, staffing issues, user acceptance, problems with the organization's strategic plan, software design, infrastructure and time management were all issues that nursing informacists listed as problems with the job (Greenwood, 2015). While nursing has been dated back since Florence Nightingale, reinventing the wheel is not something that nurses find themselves doing often. Most procedures have been completed at some point in history. Nursing informacists are considered pioneers due to the newness of this title, making trial and error or evidence-based practice how they come to learn part of their job description. Informaticist is a job description that would be ideal to a nurse [who] has used the computer software for years and can now serve as a consultant to create new software and perfect the software that is on the market now. Some nurses might even find this as a great opportunity for those that want to get off floor nursing, or work directly with patient care. Making this a highly desired retirement job, informaticists can work in management, consulting, research and academia (Decker, 2015). It also requires less manual labor, which creates a job for someone who has gotten hurt on the job and cannot perform tasks in the manner in which they were once used to. For instance, if a nurse gets hurt on the job, historically the nurse would try and work as a staff nurse if the necessary experience was acquired. Because of the increasing demand for informaticists, they can now use the experience acquired and work with software engineers to create an easier and user-friendlier computer software system.

Computer software appears to be an issue in healthcare as well. If software like Point Click Care (PCC) would become aligned with Omnicare or whatever pharmacy software used at the facility, errors could be prevented. The same software that is used for documentation is not the same software that is used for pharmacy, or for labs. The same diagnosis or orders have to be put in for the documentation, each time a medication or lab is entered. This software is available for some hospitals, but not for nursing homes and other healthcare facilities. Even the software that is used in some hospitals has been reported to have issues, or is not labeled as user friendly by most of the nurses using it. This will help nurses save more time throughout the shift, without repetitive work being completed during the shift. Also, this is an instance where if the nurse does not have basic computer skills or has problems typing, the amount of time spent on documentation, inputting orders and labs, etc. may have been increased or doubled. An example of this is a new hire nurse without necessary computer skills who spends most of his or her time at the computer inputting orders, completing documentation, inputting labs, etc. Without electronic health records (EHR), the nurse probably spends half the amount of time it takes for him or her to complete these tasks. The nurse is now spending a considerable amount of time away from the patients on the computer and is more than likely not able to complete these tasks within the shift. Some institutions may believe the nurse is "riding the clock," which threatens the nurse's job and takes time away from the nurse-patient interaction. "Riding the clock" is a term used to describe nurses who remain on the time clock while at work just to get paid for unnecessary work. They may move at a slow pace while performing tasks, when the work can be done expeditiously and can get off work in the scheduled time. This often gives the supervisor the perception that the nurse has poor time management skills and costs the institution money because labor laws require the nurse to get paid while still on the time clock. Another thing that would save time, would be the use of the same computer software universally. If hospitals, nursing homes, outpatient clinics, etc., all utilized the same system, one institution would be able to view the documentation of another without the hassle of having to call back and forth. This would save time with receiving history and with admissions, and taking reports over the phone after discharge from one facility to another. The majority of the veteran's hospitals already work using this system. Imagine how effective this process could be if this was implemented universally. It would also prevent errors when polypharmacy is involved, because pharmacies and providers everywhere would have to adopt the same software. The reasoning behind why this process has not happened is because software companies are afraid of losing money when it comes to merging. This market would and could be as lucrative as the pharmaceutical industry.

Technologically savvy nurses find themselves at an increased demand due to skills they possess to test software applications and field-test new devices. Some might even work as consultants to software developers to help build healthcare applications (Decker, 2015). For the nurse educators who are currently in the field, ignorant of computer software and applications, this becomes a threat. They have the experience necessary to teach new nurses, but find it difficult with the new computer-based work environment. This is similar to bilingual nurses who are in demand. Computers have become a second language to many. Nurses can market themselves as speaking English as well as computers. According to Westra and Delaney (2008), health information technologies (HITs) are now known as the stethoscope of the 21st century. Besides nurses' general healthcare certifications, certifications in computer software, will be required as well. This too, will cut down on the orientation time of a new nurse and similarly save time. For instance, as a new hire who is familiar with the computer system, the orientation will primarily be focused on bedside manner, rather than an introduction to computers class, thus, saving time that a nurse has to spend on orientation and [the] amount of time it takes a nurse to complete documentation in a shift. Nurse leaders are required to be competent in computer skills, but do not have to perform them. Because most leaders are not inputting documentation into EHRs, they are focused on procuring financial support for the EHR, but actually performing the task is not necessary (Westra and Delaney, 2008). One may argue that, in order to adequately teach this task, it must also be learned by the teacher. This goes along with the principle, "lead by example." Nurse educators and leaders teaching in the school and workplace environment will have to adapt or lose their titles. Essentially, the new nurses who are coming out of school are usually well versed in the use of modern healthcare with computers, making it hard for nurse educators and leaders to effectively teach without the knowledge of computers, although they have the best bedside manner.

For the next century, the study of informatics will be as fundamental to the practice of medicine as anatomy was to the last (Coiera, 1999). Informatics can be lucrative for some nurses, as a great demand is growing for this job. Finding employment in this field is easier and continues to increase. Computer software engineering companies have some work to do to make the healthcare industry run as smoothly as some of the applications used on day to day with other professions. Technologically savvy nurses have a greater advantage in healthcare than nurses who lack computer skills. Nurses who currently hold positions that supervise, manage, or educate find that the career is not secured without the necessary computer skills. Eventually, nurses without computer skills in the industry will be obsolete as they are trying to make licensed practical nurses. While this will not happen overnight, soon everyone will lean toward having an informatics officer in healthcare establishments.

References

Coiera, E. (1999). Ten essential clinical informatics skills. *Journal of the Royal Colleges of Surgeons of Edinburgh, 44*(4), 269–270. Retrieved from http://www.rcsed.ac.uk/RCSEDBackIssues/journal/vol44_4/4440042.htm

Courtney, K., Demiris, G., & Alexander, G. (2005) Information technology changing nursing processes at the point-of-care. *Journal of Nursing Administration Quarterly, 29*(4), 315–322.

Decker, F. (2015). Reasons why every nurse needs to have informatics skills. *Houston Chronicle.* Retrieved from http://work.chron.com/reasons-nurse-needs-informatics-skills-4666.html

Greenwood, B. (2015). Problems with nursing informatics. *Houston Chronicle.* Retrieved from http://work.chron.com/problems-nursing-informatics-27523.html

Marshall, S. D., Kitto, S., Shearer, W., Wilson, S. J., Finnigan, M. A., Sturgess, T., ... & Buist, M. D. (2011). Why don't hospital staff activate the rapid response system (RRS)? How frequently is it needed and can the process be improved? *Implementation Science, 6,* 39. doi:10.1186/1748-5908-6-39

Mikkelsen, G., & Aasly, J. (2001). Concordance of information in parallel electronic and paper based patient records. *International Journal of Medicine,* 123–31.

Sewell, J., & Thede, L. (2013). *Informatics and nursing: Opportunities and challenges* (4th ed.). Philadelphia, PA: Kluwer, Lippincott, Williams and Wilkins.

Smith C. A., & Haque S. N. (2006). Paper versus electronic documentation in complex chronic illness: A comparison. In American Medical Informatics Association, *Annual Symposium Proceedings* (pp. 734–738). November 11, 2006–November 15, 2006 Hilton Washington & Towers, Washington, DC

Westra, B., & Delaney, C. (2008). Informatics competencies for nursing and healthcare leaders. *AMIA Annual Symposium,* 804–808. Retrieved from http://www.ncbi.nlm.nih.gov/pmc/articles/PMC2655955

CHAPTER 2

Computer, Operating System and Software

CHAPTER HIGHLIGHTS

This chapter discusses the following:

- How computer technology has dramatically changed the way we live our everyday life, from basic activities to communicating with anyone anywhere in the world through audio and video applications information management
- How the computer is just like a piece of furniture, without the input and the software that enables the computer itself to function and application software that manages user input
- How a health are personnel who has access to or opens a patient's profile in the computer may be the single variable in protecting patient health information
- How cloud computing is differentiated from other types of hosts
- How software copyright is a form of restriction placed on software to prevent others from copying it illegally

DEFINITION

ACCORDING TO THE Oxford English dictionary, a computer is an electronic device for storing and processing data, typically in binary form, according to instructions given to it in a variable program. The first computers to be produced were bulky and slower in operation speed, but as technology has advanced and has been integrated, more efficient and smaller components have been designed.

COMPUTER USAGE AND INFORMATION MANAGEMENT

Computer technology has dramatically changed the way people live their everyday life, from basic activities such as writing and editing through word processing that checks and corrects spelling to communicating virtually with anyone, anywhere in the world through audio and video applications. The internet has made it possible to access information, upload music and photos, and learn, design, and even play games with anybody anywhere in the world. Today, travels are made easy due to the use of global positioning system (GPS), a computer communication application. Banks enable us to download their applications in conjunction with telephone carriers for easy transactions and customer satisfaction.

Information management through gathering, creating, storing, retrieving, sharing, and utilizing data has been the hallmark of nursing informatics. For an average nurse to fully understand and appreciate this revolutionary trend of computer technology, the user will have to understand the concept of information management—the tools and the technical know-how. With the introduction of electronic health records (EHR) (where patients' health records are stored, retrieved, and represented in one spot without having to track other departments for their recorded patient data), to work efficiently and improve productivity, and to maintain the pace of information technology phenomenon, it is imperative that nurses understand basic components of computer and usages. This chapter will describe some of the basic features of operating systems and how to apply basic features of operating systems, differentiate application software, define a computer algorithm, explain the importance of user group, and differentiate the various types of software copyright.

APPLICATION SOFTWARE AND INFORMATION MANAGEMENT

The computer is just a tool that accepts input, processes and stores data, and produces output. The software enables the computer itself to function, and the application software manages user input. The system software is further divided into two, the read-only memory (ROM) which is the built-in software that helps the computer to boot, and the system software known as the operating system (OS). OS is the primary software installed in PCs; it is the main software that makes it possible for all the commands to be carried out. It determines the types of applications that can be installed and manages files and software installed; it also services inputs from users by working as a middleman between users and hardware, and it breaks down the input to machine language that the hardware understands. Without the OS, the computer will not function.

According to Sewell and Thede (2013), there are different types of OS. They include Microsoft windows for most PCs, Apple Macintosh OS, Windows CE OS for PDAs, or, for hand-held devices, Palm OS. Disc-operating systems (DOS) are one of the original OS by Microsoft for PCs and are utilized based on the text and give command after text such as run, delete, and copy. The latest Microsoft OS is more user friendly than the DOS (Sewell & Thede, 2013). OS makes it possible for a user to run multiple applications at the same time and provides the ability to switch from one task to another without interruption, a function known as multitasking. OS controls all the software and hardware to run applications, share data, and boost communication.

Operating systems can be grouped into five areas as follows:

- **Multi-user OS:** Enables two or more users to run programs simultaneously without any conflict. However, some OS allows as many as hundreds or even thousands of users at same time.
- **Multiprocessing OS:** Enables the operation of a program on more than one computer.
- **Multitasking OS:** Permits more than one program to run concurrently.

- **Multithreading OS:** Permits other components of a single program to function at same time.
- **Real-time OS:** Enables input spontaneously. However, it is very important to note that DOS and UNIX, which are considered general-system OS, are not real time.

Users normally interact with the operating system through a set of commands. For example, the DOS operating system contains commands such as COPY and RENAME for copying, changing and renaming files, respectively. The commands are accepted to execute the interpretation. A graphical user interface (GUI) allows one to enter commands by pointing and clicking the desired objects that appear on the screen.

To further expand on the benefit of the OS to the learner, knowledge of the basic features of an operating system such as starting or opening and exiting the PC and knowing which button to click to access different programs and tasks will help the user to dissipate cyberphobia. It will be beneficial for nurses to understand that to begin a program, they must first click on the start button on the top left corner. A click on "All programs" opens programs for one to choose desired content. The menu bar displays all the programs and allows one to make a choice. When working on Windows, one has the choice to minimize or maximize the file by clicking the corresponding icon. The quick bar helps to move between the programs and/or files. Some other features include the mouse, which is used to point and click, copy, paste, save, cut, and print. Graphic user interfaces (GUI) are pictorial icons, which, with a click of a mouse, pick up the desired icons or pictures. If one does not know what the icon represents, one can point the mouse on the picture icon and the function of the icon will appear. GUI makes it easy to continue the flow of work when working with multiple programs without having to go back and forth. There are also security features such as log-in, password, and control access to the network. It is also important to note that OS has other hidden network monitoring functions as well as a remote control. The operating system allows basic features such as file and internet connections to occur, as well as data backup.

SOFTWARE CATEGORIES

According to research, the application software could be grouped into seven categories:

1. Internet application: This allows access to Web browsing that exposes a wide range of information. It could be accessed using common sets of communication protocol. The internet is a global electric network of computers that connect government, universities research facilities, etc. The nurse could retrieve virtually any information, including evidence-based practice from internet search engines, and customize it to fit his or her organizational needs. There is so many information on the internet, however, that the manager should try to obtain internet information from a reliable source.

2. Productivity software: This contains application programs for office work such as word processing, spread sheet creation, and database, communication, and graphic software, which can also be part of productivity. Productivity software is

among one of the reasons people buy computers. It helps the user, especially the professional, accomplish the task in efficient and superior ways than the OS alone.

3. Communication application software: This type of application facilitates talking to others through e-mailing, texting, chatting, voicemail, video, and webinar. This can be accomplished through Gmail, GMX, and chatting using applications (Sewell & Thede, 2013).

4. Graphic software: This provides basic and more complex tools that enable users to view and edit images such as photo files (point and click). Graphic software can import and export graphic files in one or more folders. It is an excellent tool for professional photographers and graphic designers. An example is the Adobe Photoshop program.

5. Multimedia programs: These assist users in the use of playing back, creating, and editing audio and video files. This multimedia combines video, radio, CD-ROMs and the internet to educate and/or entertain.

6. Game applications: This type of application exposes users to many games in the computer. More games are being introduced every so often. A person can learn to create his or her own games with the software application.

7. Utilities software: This includes antivirus, archives, backup, and screen saver software, to mention a few, but are also applications that help to remove irrelevant files from the hard drive, manage computer resources, and allow full control of the start program when one logs on (Flood, 2013).

Speech recognition is another software application used for communicating in a situation where the user is unable to use a keyboard to enter data due to certain disabilities. Instead of typing, the user may simply speak into a headset. Speech recognition requires training sessions for the computer to recognize the voice. Speech recognition software is expensive and is mostly used in rare and extreme cases. A similar computer gadget is a touch-tone screen device with a sensor on top of which a paraplegic (no motor function except his eyes, mouth, and neck) uses it to communicate. The patient eyeballs the letters, spacebar, or numbers on the screen, and the sensor types the letters. Also, if no one is in the room and the user types "nurse," another voice sensor reads and vocalizes the word to call the nurse. A paraplegic who has no use of his or her limbs or who could not speak can now type and communicate. Such is an amazing revolutionary trend of our technology world.

GROUPWARE AND PASSWORD SECURITY

Another application system is the groupware program, which

> helps people work together collectively while located remotely from each other. Programs that enable real time collaboration are called synchronous groupware, and asynchronous when they not collaborating in real time. (TechTarget, n.d.)

An example of asynchronous groupware is the wikis in text messaging, and an example of synchronous groupware is "Blackboard Collaborate" often used for distance learning.

> Groupware services can include the sharing of calendars, collective writing, e-mail handling, shared database access, electronic meetings with each person able to see and display information to others, and other activities. Groupware are sometimes called collaborative software. (TechTarget, n.d.)

An example of groupware is Microsoft Outlook where colleagues can share calendars, send each other e-mails, and communicate and schedule appointments for community healthcare workers—asynchronous groupware. Through shared calendars, the nurse leaders share scheduled appointments and/or days off with others.

According to Rouse (2010) the word application is comprised of

> a shorter form of an application program while an application program is a program designed to perform special functions directly for the user or, in some cases, for another application program. Examples of applications include word processors, web browsing, database programs, development tools, drawing, paint, image editing programs, spread sheet, and communication programs. Applications utilize the services of the computer's operating system and other supporting applications. The formal requests and means of communicating with other programs that an application program uses are called the application program interface (API). (https://whatis.techtarget.com/definition/Enterprise-Cloud-Computing-FAQ)

Finally, to exit a computer, the user must simply close all files and programs before shutting down. The shutdown button is noted on the bottom left after clicking the start button. The user must close all programs and files before shutting down the computer, otherwise the unsaved files will crowd up the hard disk that will eventually cause problems. Besides, the HIPAA law prohibits exposure of patients' information. Healthcare personnel who have access or who open a patient's profile in the computer must close the chart before exiting to prevent exposure of patient record. Another ramification of not exiting properly is others using the healthcare worker's password. Passwords are supposed to be secured in private places. They are not supposed to be shared or kept where others have access to them.

CLOUD COMPUTING

Another application worth noting is cloud computing. According to Rouse (2010), this is a term used for

> anything that involves providing hosted services over the Internet. The services are divided into three categories: Infrastructure-as-a-Service (IaaS), Platform-as-a-Service (PaaS), and Software-as-a-Service (SaaS). The name cloud computing was created from the cloud symbol that is often used to represent the Internet in flowcharts and diagrams. A cloud service has three

unique characteristics that differentiate it from other types of hosts. The characteristics are: a). It is sold on demand, b). It is typically by the minute or the hour; c). It is elastic—a user can have as much or as little of a service as they want at any given time; and d). The service is fully managed by the host provider. The consumer needs nothing other than the personal computer and Internet access. (Rouse, 2010, https://whatis.techtarget.com/definition/Enterprise-Cloud-Computing-FAQ)

Cloud computing is in high demand due to innovations in virtualization, improved access to high-speed internet, a weak economy, and distributed computing. Algorithms are sets of instructional flow charts in computer language. They are used to explain step-by-step processes of plans. They are a set of rules or queries that a programmer uses to solve problems in as few steps as possible. Basic algorithms are comprised of letters, zeros, and straight bars or the numeric 1. Some of the programming language includes COBOL, FORTRA, R and so forth. Algorithms are not used for basic input and output, rather they are used for more complex and sophisticated problems in computer programming. An example is the algorithm that recognizes software code or product number during software registration (Sewell & Thede, 2013).

SOFTWARE PIRACY AND COPYRIGHT PROTECTION

Again, the importance of user groups cannot be overemphasized. User groups are organized users of typical forms of hardware and software products. The makeup of user groups may range from novice nurses to computer programming consultants. There are internal and external groups. Members meet to share ideas and experiences to improve their understanding and use of the product. User groups are often responsible for influencing vendors to modify or enhance their product. For internal groups, nurses from different department are encouraged to participate to contribute, learn, and share best practices that benefit their colleagues.

Software copyright is a form of restriction placed on the software to prevent others from copying the software illegally. Kinds of copyrights include proprietary, shareware, freeware, or public domain copyrights. Proprietary copyrights, such as Microsoft, believe that selling software indirectly represents purchasers buying licenses to use the software. So, they dubbed the agreement between the proprietor and purchaser as an end-user license agreement (EULA). In this sense, the proprietor or manufacturer requires purchasers to register the product to use the internet. In the process, certain product numbers, called serial numbers or product keys that come with the software, are registered for product identification purposes. For example, Microsoft will check number to see if the product had been registered before it will be registered again. This is their way of checking copyright.

Another type of copyright is the shareware. The distributors of the software encourage distribution of the software during a trial period for free, but ask that users pay some money after they try the product and like it. This is an indirect way of advertising as well as sharing. Freeware is the other type of copyright. The programmer allows free use of the application and at same time decides when it is to be used. Public domain is an example of freeware such as the internet. Anyone can access any information in the internet. Users can copy, alter, and use this information without any restrictions. It is highly encouraged to check for virus content using an antiviral tool before downloading and storing such information.

> Most software programs purchased are licensed for use by just one user or at just one computer site. Moreover, when someone buys software, he or she is known as a "licensed user" rather than as an owner of the software. As a licensed user, an individual is permitted to make copies of the software program for back-up purposes only. It is a violation of copyright laws in North America, in particular, to freely distribute software copies. Because software piracy is all but impossible to halt entirely, software companies now launch legal suits against individuals violating software copyright laws. Years ago, software companies attempted to prevent software piracy by copy-protecting software, but this strategy was neither foolproof nor convenient for users. Software companies typically require registration at the time of software purchase in an attempt to clamp down on the problem. (Schell & Martin, 2010)

Unauthorized copying of some purchased software describes software theft, and is punishable by law. The copyright protection bill was passed by Congress in 1998 and is called the Digital Millennium Copyright Act (DMCA). It was enacted to protect illegal copying of software. The offense ranges from misdemeanor to felony and carries up to $100,000 for statutory damages and $250,000 for the crime. To avoid the heavy fine and/or risking jail time, it is imperative to abide by the manufacturers' decisions and processes of copyright.

The days of long, tedious, and time-consuming manual data entry and computing are gone. The evolving computer technology had made the world figuratively small; an individual could chart, play games, and obtain information across the globe within a fraction of time, but it took years to reach this milestone. With the evolution of computer technology, some older ways of communicating, such as typewriting and telegramming, are now being replaced by more efficient and time-saving computer technology such as word processing, e-mailing, Skyping, EHR, and webinar. Computer technology has also enhanced multitasking. Knowledge of software information management will boost nurses' confidence and assist them in thriving in this technology-driven market place.

Student Experience: Computer Operating System

Allison Martin, RN, BSN

In a world where computers, cell phones, iPods, phablets, TVs, and tablets are commonplace, each of these devices uses an operating system. According to Dictionary.com, "The operating system is a collection of software that directs a computer's operations, controlling and scheduling the execution of other programs, and managing storage, input/output, and communication resources" (2015). In a nutshell, the operating system is the most important program on the computer (Sewell & Thede, 2013, p. 22). Without an operating system, the electronic device is practically an expensive paperweight.

Due to cost and ease of use, many personal computers come pre-installed with and use a version of Microsoft Windows operating systems. Microsoft Windows is a graphical user interface (GUI) that enables the user to point and click icons to enact commands instead of typing them. For this reason, many healthcare systems use a version of Microsoft Windows for their computer systems (Sewell & Thede, 2013, p. 22).

There have been several versions of Windows operating systems released between the years of 1990–2015. The version timeline for some of the Windows personal operating systems are as follows: Windows 3.0, Windows 3.1, Windows 95, Windows 98, Windows Me, Windows XP, Windows Vista, Windows 7, Windows 8, Windows 8.1, and Windows 10 (Microsoft, 2013). The student has had the opportunity to use each of these versions. It is generally thought that with each new Windows updated version, the operating system makes computing easier for the user. However, as it was discovered over the years, some versions caused more challenges and complaints than usual. The three that were disliked the most were Windows Me, Windows Vista, and Windows 8. Windows XP and Windows 7 were the favorites. Windows 10 is too new for there to be a general consensus on whether it is a good or bad operating system as of yet.

Windows Me, released in 1999, was designed for home use, introducing music and video playback, in addition to movie making. These features were nice, but the operating system did not seem sound or stable. Unfortunately, over time, the system would hang regularly and required regular reboots. It was also prone to getting viruses. On a good note, it had system restore; the system could be rolled back to a date or time before a system problem occurred. However, this feature was used continuously and too frequently to be able to repair regular roll backs. It was time again for a new Windows operating system. Users were happy when Windows XP was released.

Released in 2001, Windows XP was a beloved operating system that became one of the best-selling Microsoft products (Microsoft, 2013). Windows XP was a stable and fast operating system. It provided greater access to online help and support features. This operating system was well-planned and delivered sound functionality to users. Windows XP users had a sound operating system that they could trust for many years. In 2015, there were many that are still using the Windows XP operating system, despite it being outdated and prone to security breaches. Internet Explorer and certain browsers with added security features are not compatible anymore with Windows XP. Windows XP users will eventually have to upgrade to another operating system.

Windows Vista was introduced in 2006 to counter the growing security threats from viruses in emails, programs, and media on Windows XP. Windows Vista was an operating system with increased security measures that asked the user for permission for every task. This was a cumbersome feature to approve a security measure with each program or file opened. The system was more secure, but Windows Vista locked up every application and task. Users eventually got used to it; however, there was such an outcry about how bad Windows Vista was, Microsoft eventually offered the chance to go back to XP. Many users took that option. After that, many users were reluctant to try new versions of Windows, despite upgrades in security and functionality.

To quell some of the complaints about Windows Vista, Microsoft marketed Windows 7 as "a better version of Windows XP." There were several reasons why many people liked the Windows 7 operating system and continue to use it. It was very similar to Windows XP, but with added security measures and program stability. It is easy to find programs, files, and information when needed. It works well with plug-ins, most printers, and educational software. Users were able to use it immediately, without out any instruction. The student will continue to use Windows 7 on other computers owned.

Windows 10 was recently released in August 2015 to counter the many complaints Microsoft received regarding Windows 8. Problems included how to control active tiles, the lack of the start button, taking longer to find files and programs, and the touch screen interface. Windows 8 was an operating system that was supposed to work both on cell phones and on home computers. Users embraced the system for their phones and tablets. However, it was not a welcomed change for their home computers. In order to get more consumers to be receptive to the new Windows 10 operating system quickly, Microsoft offered free upgrades to those who owned Windows 7 and Windows 8.1. These two systems were chosen as they allowed for the least amount of computer system upgrades for the update. For the first time in Microsoft history, a free and full version of a Windows operating system was being offered to eligible owners (Microsoft, 2015). Since Windows XP users are diehard supporters, it was questioned why the upgrade would not be offered to them. It would have made sense to offer the upgrade to entice them to convert (M. McArthur, personal communication, September 4, 2015). However, Microsoft's response stated that the computers that were still running Windows XP would not be able to run Windows 10 properly (Microsoft, 2015). According to an article in TechRadar.pro, most Windows 7 users will continue to use it, instead of upgrading to Windows 10 (Galindo, 2014). This is due to the fact that there are not many features that have changed between the two systems.

This computer originally came pre-installed with the Microsoft Windows 7 operating system. Windows 7 was released in 2009 (Microsoft, 2013). It is easy to use with a seamless operating system. The student was very comfortable using this operating system. Programs, files, and system settings were easy to locate and use. It also worked well with other web browsers and software. Since a Windows operating system is usually offered every four years, the student considered upgrading for a future computer. She was very aware of the issues with Windows 8 and wanted to wait until Windows 10 was released for new systems. When the alert came to upgrade to the new operating system Windows 10 for free on this computer, the student grappled with whether or not to upgrade. There was skepticism that Microsoft was giving away free, full versions of the newest operating system. For Microsoft to do this was unheard of. Microsoft is one of the highest grossing software companies in the world. Many questions were being asked about the new software release. Something must be wrong with it if Microsoft is giving the full version of an operating system for free. Was it a good update? Would it cause too many problems during installation? Would it be compatible with current software and hardware? What happens if it does not work with the computer? The student took the plunge and recently upgraded to the new operating system Windows 10 on [her] computer. So far, the student has been pleased with the update. There are some components of Windows 8 included in Windows 10. A variation of the tile system is included. It is a little hard to find the control panel when doing a search of the computer. There were some things that required adjusting to, but not enough to want to uninstall.

As many healthcare facilities currently use, the student's hospital also uses Windows 7 as the operating system of choice. For the past six years prior to April 2014, the hospital had been using Windows XP. This system would probably still be used if it had not been dropped from customer and technical support by Microsoft. Luckily, due to the similarities to Windows XP, hospital personnel have been able to transition to the newer operating system without disruption in researching medications, patient charting, and printing admission and discharge paperwork. This is a great thing in continuing to provide excellent care to patients. Also, there are classes being offered to those personnel who need more help in navigating the system.

References

Dictionary.com. (2015). *Operating system*. Retrieved from http://dictionary.reference.com/browse/operating system

Flood, C. (2013). *What is the meaning of computer software?*. Retrieved from https://www.outsystems.com/cpc/native-vs-web-vs-hybrid/?utm_source=google&utm_medium=cpc&utm_campaign=Low%20Priority%20-%20USA%20-%20NA&utm_term=%2Bweb%20%2Bapp&utm_content=Low%20Priority_Web%20App_BRO&gclid=CjwKCAjw7cDaBRBtEiwAsxprXUy_YfFCQxUmKGZEPBbKAlGWhze6AVji7xu0kqr8ipZCGy3EWiUHi-RoCwYMQAvD_

Galindo, S. (2014). Will Windows 10 be the catalyst for the remaining Windows XP users to upgrade?. *TechRadar*. Retrieved from http://www.techradar.com/us/news/software/operating-systems/will-windows-10-be-the catalyst-for-the-remaining-windows-xp-users-to-upgrade--1270027

Microsoft. (2013). *A history of Windows*. Retrieved from http://windows.microsoft.com/en-US/windows/history#T1=era10

Microsoft. (2015). *Windows 10 FAQ and tips*. Retrieved from http://www.microsoft.com/en-US/windows/windows-10-faq

Rouse, M. (2010). SaaS applications integration: Strategies and best practices for success. Retrieved from https://whatis.techtarget.com/definition/Enterprise-Cloud-Computing-FAQ

Schell, B. & Martin, M. (2010). Webster's new world hacker dictionary. Hoboken, NJ: Wiley.

Sewell, J. P., Thede, L. Q., & Thede, L. Q. (2013). Software: Information management. In *Informatics and nursing: Opportunities and challenges* (4th ed.) (pp. 21–33). Philadelphia, PA: Lippincott Williams & Wilkins.

TechTarget. (n.d.). *Groupware*. Retrieved from https://searchdomino.techtarget.com/definition/groupware

CHAPTER 3

Computer Networks, Applications, Concerns, and Security Measures

CHAPTER HIGHLIGHTS

This chapter discusses the following:

- How a system of interlinked computers' exchange information to and from each other as in LAN and WAN networks
- How computer systems that are used in most health facilities function by communicating through a main server
- How World Wide Web (also coined W3 or WWW) is just a portion of the larger internet and sometimes interchangeably confused
- How online security is a major concern for anyone who utilizes a computer network that connects to the internet and measures to combat such malicious activities
- Student's perspective on *"Effects of the Internet on Society and Healthcare"*

According to Apter, (2010),

> Clinical Nurse Specialists (CNSs) interested in the effects of technology on nursing practice and patient care have a great opportunity to make improved changes in practice and the environment where they work through the creative use of technology. The informatics CNS is important to make sure that nurses embrace information technologies in support of practice. An informatics CNS with clinical experience and informatics skills could be an asset in a healthcare institution. Such a position in addition, is strategically positioned as the best insurance for successful use of health information technologies. This role can support nurses and be made available in the management of information systems. As healthcare organizations are being rapidly transitioned to an electronic health record, a CNS with competencies in informatics can be instrumental to nurses and other disciplines requiring technologies to support their daily activities in practice. This unique role could also enable healthcare professionals like nurses to use information to enhance health delivery and effectiveness. (Apter, 2010)

LAN AND WAN CONCEPTS

COMPUTER NETWORKS, ALSO interchanged with data networks, are systems of interlinked computers that exchange information to and from each other. The established networks are known as links and the computer devices that communicate the information are known as nodes. The internet is a well-known example of how these networks function. Networks vary in size and in location. The two most-used types of networks are the local area networks (LAN) or the wide area networks (WAN). The local area networks are those that users most likely deal with on a day-to-day basis in different practice areas. These comprise a series of computers that are geographically close in proximity. Wide area networks are very similar to LAN. Wide area networks are also a series of computers that are interlined but usually cover a much larger geographic area and consist of multiple LANs.

CLIENT/SERVER TYPE

There are many different variations to make up the virtual infrastructure of computer networks. The two most common types are peer to peer and client/server type. The peer-to-peer variation is that of a home computer. It is not connected to another computer and stands alone in its functioning. The second type of client server is one with which most nurses are familiar. These are the computer systems that are used in most health facilities and function by communicating through a main server. Beyond making the initial request, rarely is any of this process visible to the user (Sewell & Thede, 2013). As there is a structure of virtually linked computer networks, there is also the means by which they are physically connected. A hard-wired or permanent connection uses materials such as phone lines, fiber optic cables, or radio waves. Wireless connectivity (Wi-Fi) also utilizes "hard" connections but transmits on a limited scale through nodes that are placed throughout a building. The network nodes components originate, route, and terminate the data.

CONNECTION SETUP

Nodes are comprised of hosts such as servers and personal computers and are networking hardware inclusive. In a wireless-type connection setup, nodes are placed in specific locations to transmit the most optimal signal. The nodes pick up the signal sent by a user and relay this information back to a central process or the originator's computer. Since security is one of the major concerns with a wireless network, there are measures that can be employed to protect information transmitted over them. Wired-equivalent privacy and Wi-Fi protected access were created to reduce these security risks. To set up a wireless network, one must first have a broadband internet connection with a digital subscriber line or a cable modem, a wireless router, and a computer with wireless network capabilities (Sewell & Thede, 2013).

For networks to operate optimally, it is imperative that there be an effective exchange of communication known as protocols. The transmission control protocol/internet protocol (TCP/IP) is the basic language of the internet. It allows for the interoperable transmission of data on the internet. To use the internet and the Web, there must first be a connection to a computer network. This interaction allows for joint use of software or hardware applications and devices (Wink, 2009). It is a known fact that access to the internet is obtained through an internet service provider. Connection to the internet through the internet service provider can occur in several different ways. Two of those ways to connect are through telephone service (POTS) or broadband service. The availability of these services is dependent on factors such as geographical area and distance from the service provider. The speed of the connection is determined by type of connection and internet service provider (ISP).

The four main types of broadband connection from fastest to slowest are fiber optic cable, television cable, satellite, and digital subscriber lines. Fiber optic cable is the fastest means of transmitting data. It carries data over a cable line, which is composed of glass, in the form of light. Due to its delicate glass structure, it also makes it the most expensive means of providing internet service. Conversely, it is the most durable. Cable connections are similar in functioning to that of DSL to a telephone line in that they utilize portions of the cable line to transmit data. It does not interfere with television service nor does it require the television to be operating at time of use. Satellite usually incurs a higher cost to set up than cable due to the requirement of an antenna. Another drawback to satellite is the interference of service in severe weather conditions and built-in delay reception because the signal has to travel a significant distance. Digital subscriber lines (DSL) use telephone lines to transmit data and require a special line split tool to allow use of DSL service and phone service simultaneously without interruption. Although it is the slowest of all broadband connections, it is faster than Plain Old Telephone Service (POTS) that most homes use. In contrast, the telephone services based on high-speed, digital communications lines, such as ISDN and FDDI, are not POTS. The differences between POTS and non-POTS services are speed and bandwidth. It is important to note that POTS is generally restricted to about 52 Kbps (52,000 bits per second).

> To date, most residential customers to the internet have used dial-up modems with a top speed of about 56.6 kbps [kilobits per second]. Broadband access has become available via digital subscriber lines (DSL) offered by the local regulated telephone company. Cable modems and DSL offer access speeds about 10–30 times higher than dial up access and termed "broadband Internet access." (Hausman, 2001)
>
> In addition to broadband and dial-up services, web users are now able to connect to the internet wirelessly. This permits access to the web without wires or cables of any type. Wireless technology allows users to have mobile connections, accessing the web (with some limitations) where and when they need to. This can be accomplished via public Wi-Fi networks, cellular services, and Wimax — a somewhat newer type of wireless service. Access is available anytime, anywhere, as long as you are connected to the Internet and have access to a Web browser. (Wink, 2009)

INTERNET AND WORLD WIDE WEB (WWW)

The internet is a global network of interlinked computers. It has grown substantially in the past 20 years and has become quickly assimilated into daily use (Sewell & Thede, 2013). The World Wide Web (also coined W3 or WWW) is just a portion of the larger internet and sometimes interchangeably confused. It was created as a means to sustain communication in the event of nuclear war. Much of the internet's growth and success is due to its free and open access, sometimes termed "net neutrality."

> The exponential growth of the World-Wide Web has transformed it into an ecology of knowledge in which highly diverse information is linked in an extremely complex and arbitrary manner. (Reka, Hawoong, & Albert-Laszlo, 1999)

Also, the number of websites has been growing exponentially since its inception, which means that there are many more young sites than old ones. The World Wide Web is often times viewed as a huge online library. At the tap of a few keys or click of a few buttons, an individual will have access to an infinite amount of information on any given subject and at any given time. On the other hand, scrutiny must be used when evaluating information obtained from the Web because anyone can obtain a website and post anything.

A Web browser is the medium used to access this information. The home page is the initial page that pops open when accessing the browser. Navigating through a Web document or scrolling up and down can be performed either using your mouse or your four arrow keys. Use of the mouse is usually easier to maneuver when thumbing through a page, especially if accessing a hyperlink (hot area) to continue on to a new web page. Just as individual computers have addresses to identify their location, called IP addresses, documents posted on the Web possess them as well. The address allows for direct access to that specific page and consists of a computer name and domain name, contains no spaces, only utilizes forward slashes, and is often case sensitive. In previous years, domain names were only three letters long and could help decipher what type of organization was sponsoring that particular page. Due to the international growth of Web involvement, it has now been expanded to up to 63 characters. For convenience, Web browsers allow for the use of either a favorites or bookmarks tab. This tab will save some of the most visited sites and allow for quicker future access to them. The internet also allows for the exchange of information, not only in text but also in the form of audio and video. Streaming of audio and video will allow for the use of the material being accessed before it has even had the opportunity to be fully downloaded.

World Wide Web technology is also comparatively used as a private network among institutions. This intranet is a closed network that allows for an efficient and cost-effective way for information to be shared within an agency by many subscribers to specific information at one time. Because it is a closed network, the information published on the intranet cannot be accessed by the outside world. Although, it is still possible for subscribers inside an institution to have access to both the internet and intranet. Another use of WWW technology is an extranet. This basically allows for external access to a company's intranet by individuals not physically inside an institution. It allows this access through user name and password.

ONLINE SECURITY CONCERNS AND PROTECTION MEASURES

There are some things to watch out for online. Online security is a major concern for anyone who utilizes a computer network that connects to the internet. Malware, also known as malicious software, includes viruses and spyware that get installed on the computer or mobile device without the users' knowledge. Malware is created by criminals to steal personal information, interfere with the operations of a computer system, and perform fraudulent tasks. Malware is intended to do harm; however, there are other reasons for malware, such as to gather information from government and corporate websites.

There are four key types of malware to consider, and these are sometimes also referred to as the four horsemen: spam, bugs, denials of service, and malicious software. Spam is defined as unwanted junk mail usually sent out in bulk. Bugs are software problems that slowly evolve and can kill the computer's software. Denials of service will steal a portion of the computers resources, such as the memory, which may cause a complete system shut down. Lastly, there is malicious software that covers a wide variety of threats including botnets, viruses, worms, Trojan horses, adware, and spyware. Boatnets are a series of internet-linked computers that have become overrun by a virus or worm. A computer virus is the most commonly heard-about type of malware. This malware type copies itself into other computer programs and files without the knowledge of the computer operator. It can be contracted by something as simple as downloading an audio or music file or opening an e-mail attachment. Unlike plain virus or an e-mail virus, worms do not attach themselves to the program. However, they always cause harm to a network, even if only consuming bandwidth (Sewell & Thede, 2013). The Trojan horse is intended to operate similarly to the wooden Trojan horse in ancient Greek mythology. It mimics a legitimate piece of software to get access to the computer's operating system. Adware serves to produce revenue for the program writer. It allows for pop-up advertisements while connected to the internet. Spyware monitors Web activity and surfing to cater advertisements toward the user. It also has the ability to monitor key strokes, thus keeping record of sensitive information. It can also make changes within the user's computer.

The degree of damage by viruses varies by type of malware. Malicious software poses the greatest threat, and although phishing and pharming are older forms of scams related to the Web, they continue to pose a threat as well. Phishing and pharming both operate to obtain the user's personal information by acting as a Web address imposter, then requiring an account confirmation. This is usually achieved through a link that is e-mailed to a subscriber requesting a password or account change that will force the e-mailer to expose this information. Lastly, there are the empty threats to operating systems through hoaxes and urban legends. Hoaxes are created to fool people into thinking that there is a virus attached to an e-mail and usually require the recipient to forward the message to everyone's contact list to avoid contracting the virus. Sometimes these hoaxes scare individuals into deleting important files off their computer to avoid that virus, thus creating a major system operation problem.

There are many measures that can be taken to protect computers and prevent such malicious activity. One simple measure is utilizing secure Web pages, denoted by the lock icon or "https," when personal or sensitive information is to be transmitted. Frequent clearing of Web cookies is also important. Web cookies typically store information such as passwords for ease and convenience that can later become quite dangerous and pose as a potential risk if tracked. One must also take caution in the information that is downloaded and crosscheck the reliability of websites. If the site appears suspicious, then it is best to exit or close the site immediately. A user must refrain from using another individual's universal serial bus (USB) drive or device. If you must use it, then scan it with some type of security software. Once a computer is infected with a virus, there is anti-virus software that can be downloaded to assist with the removal of the harmful item. This software provides real-time protection to the computer. It is important to keep it updated and set up to scan the computer automatically on a regular basis and to look for patterns that may indicate an infection. This process can take up to 4 hours, so it should most likely be scheduled at a time when the device will be out of use.

In conclusion, computers and its technology are still relatively new when compared to other widely used technologies. It has evolved over the past decades and continues to grow rapidly each day. With the development of faster, sleeker, and more portable devices, this activity will continue to feed and fuel today's technology-hungry society. Global reaches of the internet, e-mail, and the World Wide Web are unprecedented. Connection speeds to the internet continue to increase. Knowledge is now more easily obtained and shared amongst the entire world. Organizations, especially acute care hospital settings and educational institutions, have come to know the benefit of the growth of computer technology over the past 5 to 10 years, especially in the face of the development and implementation of electronic medical records and the rise in college-level online learning opportunities. Consequently, the mal-intent of individuals desiring to use this technology to damage others has also grown. Viruses and malware continue to pose everyday serious threats to patrons of the internet. Thankfully, with ongoing technological advancements and development, effective means of protecting against threats are readily available. These advancements serve to greatly reduce or eliminate risk of damages associated with malware. As society continues to flourish in its embrace of the internet, computers, networks, and technology as essential in daily life, users must also remain mindful of cyber threats with the same level of vigor.

Student's Experience: Effects of the Internet on Society and Healthcare

Mekonnem Magdawit, RN, BSN

Technology and communication considerably influence society in a variety of ways, especially through the availability of knowledge and information. People can communicate rapidly and effectively with other people from around the world due to the internet. Rapid communication considerably influences the interrelationships between the members of society. Social media websites also influence the values, perceptions, and beliefs of many people primarily due to interaction with people from other cultures and nationalities. The abundance of knowledge on the internet significantly enhanced the awareness of users, especially with respect to professional terminologies, processes, and functions (Wang, 2015). However, the internet also amplified the dissemination of false or incorrect information about a variety of topics or subjects. The internet enabled people to access a plethora of knowledge and information relevant to various aspects of society, including healthcare. This paper analyzes and explains the effects of rapid communication and availability of knowledge through the internet on society and healthcare.

Rapid communication and the internet shape the perceptions, beliefs, and values of people in the context of specific settings, including healthcare. The increased interaction of people through the internet has led to a decreased level of interpersonal interactions and relationships. People usually prefer to interact and communicate with others through technological means rather than personal interactions (Celik, et al., 2014). On the other hand, the plethora of knowledge available on the internet also influences people to access information about specialized subjects through the internet. Many people read articles, website pages, and other digital material for specific issues rather than consulting with professionals and experts (Damnjanovic et al., 2015). For example, many people attempt to seek and implement cures or remedies for their ailments through the internet rather than visiting doctors. Although the internet provides significant information relevant to healthcare, experts and professionals are vital for diagnosing and treating diseases in an effective manner. On the other hand, the internet and rapid communications also allow healthcare professionals and patients to interact and communicate in an efficient manner.

The rapid communication and availability of knowledge via the internet considerably affects the interaction between patients and healthcare providers, including nurses. The availability of information and knowledge on the internet enable nurses and healthcare practitioners to teach and guide patients in an effective manner. The internet also allows nurses to evaluate the recent advancements in nursing along with the introduction of new treatment alternatives. Nurses can guide or teach patients regarding alternative treatment options in the context of recent advancements and developments in healthcare. Nurses can also help patients understand the appropriate lifestyle changes and adjustments required for chronic or acute diseases through the internet. The nurses or other healthcare practitioners can guide patients to use appropriate and credible internet sources to review several aspects of specific diseases (Kalckreuth, Trefflich, & Rummel, 2014). Rapid communications also allow nurses to convey important information to patients or their relatives in an effective manner.

Nurses can also help patients or their families to make important decisions relevant to treatment alternatives by utilizing useful internet websites. Conversely, patients can also access important data and information to understand the causes, diagnoses, treatments, and courses of actions for specific diseases. One of the most prominent influences of the internet with respect to the nursing profession is increased awareness of the patients. The increased awareness of patients regarding medical conditions and diseases enables them to make informed decisions regarding treatment options (Walsh, Hamilton, White, & Hyde, 2015). Nurses can also reduce the incidents of negative emotions and negative reactions of patients by utilizing communication channels in an effective manner (Lee & Wei, 2015). The abundance of data and information available on the internet along with a variety of communication mediums affect the attitudes and beliefs of people. Nurses can enhance their knowledge regarding appropriate methods of care and healthcare service delivery by analyzing recent trends in communications.

Developing personal and effective relationships with patients is one of the most important components of the philosophy of nursing. The availability of multiple communication channels along with technological devices also allows nurses to develop effective relationships with patients. The beliefs, expectations, and attitudes of patients stem from their cultural, racial, ethnic, and religious associations. The cultural diversity of modern society involves a variety of perceptions and views regarding healthcare due to cultural differences. Nurses need to understand the beliefs, expectations, attitudes, values, and perceptions of patients regarding healthcare services and treatments. Nurses and other healthcare practitioners can understand the expectations of patients regarding healthcare services and treatment options. The availability of knowledge on the internet regarding cultural perceptions allows nurses to understand the expectations and needs of patients in an effective manner (Bujnowska, 2015).

The internet and social media both in the current era are playing an important role in the overall development of healthcare (Iudicissa & Oliveri, 1997). Utilizing social media is a common norm these days and several hospitals utilize different benefits of social media to convey general health related information. Practitioners can convey personalized help through social media websites in an effective manner. Hospitals can provide not just basic healthcare news, but they can also provide general information about the hospital so that people can attain beneficial results from this perspective (Kotenko, 2013). However, privacy infringement can be a downside of this approach, as doctors cannot post a reply publicly. Muddling of social relationships between doctors, nurses and patients through this platform can take place.

Several websites post healthcare content online and people can easily review these websites. People can learn about different diseases and their general cure. However, a negative perspective might occur that people might determine for self-medication, and this might result in serious consequences. (Krotoski, 2011).

Advantages of this rapid communication would focus on the effective implementation of technological factors that would benefit the general healthcare. However, affordability would play an effective role in this regard, as several people might not be able to afford such newly formed technological resources. This would increase the burden on patients, as doctors would urge the patients to opt for technologically enhanced options. Nurses and other related staff would benefit in this regard. Different nurses on the other hand have to learn new methodologies because they cannot work with the same old ideologies. They have to mold themselves according to different new methodologies that would benefit the entire healthcare system in the longer run. Internet can be beneficial for general individuals too, but self-medication can act as a counter argument in this scenario. Individuals who are unable to afford the expenses might opt for different natural options from the internet. The authenticity of such options might create problems for these individuals in the long run.

Nurses and different healthcare providers have to focus on different technology oriented perspectives. They have to change their general procedure of work and learn new methodologies. Nurses should learn new communicational perspectives, as it is possible that they have to communicate with their patients through internet. In a broader perspective, nurses and different related staff have to learn how they can communicate with the implementation of effective technological outcomes. Learning new software, email procedures, textual matters, information searching, etc. would benefit them in their overall careers.

Conclusively, the internet and different social media platforms influence the social norms in an effective manner. However, they can be negative at times, and it all depends on ... whether people and medical doctors implement them in an effective manner or not. Although these aspects affect societal norms, they have changed the general outlook of the healthcare system. Nurses should learn new technologies, and higher and health institutions should train them in an effective manner, so that they can implement these ideologies in a proactive manner. A change agent can play a viable role in this regard. Change agents can teach the benefits and drawbacks of internet-based applications to different individuals of healthcare. Organizations should also consider the cost of these perspectives because they might falter in the end if they are not sure about the cost associated with these scenarios.

References

Apter, J. (2010). Informatics nurse specialist role: Integrating technology into practice [Abstract]. *Clinical Nurse Specialist, 24*(2), 97. doi:10.1097/01.NUR.0000348939.60210.39

Bujnowska, F. M. (2015). Trends in the use of the Internet for health purposes in Poland. *BMC Public Health, 15*(1), 1–17.

Celik, B., Ones, K., Celik, E. C., Bugdayci, D. S., Paker, N., Avci, C., ... (2014). The effects of using the Internet on the health-related
quality of life in people with spinal cord injury: A controlled study. *Spinal Cord, 52*(5), 388–391.

Damnjanovic, I., Kitic, D., Stefanovic, N., Zlatkovic, G. S., Catic, D. A., & Velickovic, R. R. (2015). Herbal self-medication use in patients with Diabetes Mellitus Type 2. *Turkish Journal of Medical Sciences, 45*(4), 964–971.

Hausman, J. (2001). Mismeasured variables in econometric analysis: Problems from the right and problems from the left. *Journal of Economic Perspectives, 15*(4), 57–67. doi:10.1257/jep.15.4.57

Iudicissa, S., & Oliveri, N. (1997). *Internet, telematics and health.* Amsterdam; Washington, D.C.: IOS Press; Tokyo: Ohmsha. Retrieved from https://www.worldcat.org/title/internet-telematics-and-health/oclc/37388719

Kalckreuth, S., Trefflich, F., & Rummel, K. C. (2014). Mental health related Internet use among psychiatric patients: A cross-sectional analysis. *BMC Psychiatry, 14*(1), 1–25.

Kotenko, J. (2013, April 18). The doctor will see you now: How the Internet and social media are changing healthcare. *Digital Trends.* Retrieved from http://www.digitaltrends.com/social-media/the-internet-and-healthcare/

Krotoski, A. (2011, January 9). What effect has the internet had on healthcare? *The Guardian.* Retrieved from http://www.theguardian.com/technology/2011/jan/09/untangling-web-krotoski-health-nhs

Lee, Y. C., & Wei, L. W. (2015). Effects of medical disputes on Internet communications of negative emotions and negative online word-of-mouth. *Psychological Reports, 177*(1), 251–270.

Reka, A., Hawoong, J., & Albert-Laszlo, B. (1999, September 9). Diameter of the World Wide Web. *Nature, 401*, 130–131. Retrieved from http://barabasi.com/f/65.pdf.

Sewell, J. P., & Thede, L. Q. (2013). *Informatics and nursing* (4th ed.). Philidelphia, PA: Lippincott Williams & Wilkins.

Walsh, A. M., Hamilton, K., White, K. M., & Hyde, M. K. (2015). Use of online health information to manage children's health care: A prospective study investigating parental decisions. *BMC Health Services Research, 15*(1), 1–10.

Wang, R. (2015). Internet use and the building of social capital for development: A network perspective. *Information Technologies & International Development, 11*(2), 19–34.

Wink, D. (2009). Teaching with technology computer basics. *Nurse Educator, 34*(1), 3–5.

UNIT II

CHAPTER 4

An Overview of Nursing Informatics

CHAPTER HIGHLIGHTS

This chapter discusses the following:

- How the new nursing specialty is still involving, as there is no definitive agreement on what nursing informatics means to date
- How nursing informatics is designed to improve nursing documentation, which can be used to expand knowledge, which in turn translates to quality healthcare
- How new technological shifts of the healthcare industry have improved exponentially, creating healthier patients and more competent nurses due to less stress with a decreased workload
- How the new development in other areas, such as in distance teaching and evidenced-based research, has drastically affected the role of healthcare professionals, academia, and researchers

NURSING INFORMATICS BEING DEFINED

HEALTHCARE INFORMATION IS focused on health information management. It is an umbrella term that describes the capture and storage of information. The use of information technology (IT) in healthcare is known as informatics and it is focused on information management, not merely the use of computers. Informatics is about managing healthcare information. The tendency to relate it to computers comes from the fact that the ability to manage large amounts of information is associated with computer. It also progressed as computers became more powerful and common place. Informatics originated from a Russian term "informatica." There is still no definitive agreement on what nursing informatics means because this new nursing specialty is still involving. However, over the years, Sewell and Thede from 1999–2013 have systematically and scholarly compiled "nursing informatics" definitions as enumerated in the following link http://dlthede.net/informatics/chap01introni/ni_definitions.html.

- **Sackett and Erdley (2002):** "The discipline of science which investigates the structures and properties (not specific content) of scientific information ..." (Collen (1995) as cited in Sackett & Erdley).
- **Francois Gremy** is credited with coining the term *informatique medical*, translated to medical informatics (Hannah, Ball & Edwards, 1999): "the informational

technologies which are concerned with patient care and the medical decision-making process. Another definition stated that medical informatics is the complex data processing by the computer to create new information."

- **Scholes and Barber** in 1980 in their address to the MEDINFO conference that year in Tokyo: "Health-care Informatics, however, is truly interdisciplinary. In its truest form it focuses on the care of the patient, not a specific discipline (Hannah, Ball, & Edwards, 1999). Thus, although there are specific bodies of knowledge for each healthcare profession, nursing, dentistry, dietetics, pharmacy, medicine, etc., they interface at the patient."
- **Hannah (1985):** "The use of information technology in relation to any of the functions which are within the purview of nursing and which are carried out by nurses. Hence, any use of information technology by nurses in relation to the care of patients, or the educational preparation of individuals to practice in the discipline is considered nursing informatics." (p. 181)
- **Peterson and Gerdin-Jelger (1988):** *Preparing nurses for using information systems: Recommended informatic competencies.* Published by National League for Nursing, LN Pub No. 14-2234. ISBN-13: 978-0887374166. They gave examples which included using artificial intelligence or decision-making systems, computerized scheduling, computer-assisted learning for patients or nursing education, a hospital information systems of research.
- **Graves & Corcoran (1989):** "A combination of computer science, information science, and nursing science designed to assist in the managements and processing of nursing data, information, and knowledge to support the practice of nursing and the delivery of nursing care." (p. 227)
- **McGonigle & Eggers (1991):** "The synthesis of nursing science, information management science, and computer science to enhance the input, retrieval, manipulation and/or distribution of nursing data." (p. 194).
- **ANA Council on Computer Applications in Nursing (1992):** "[A] specialty that integrates nursing science, computer science, and information science in identifying, collecting, processing, and managing data and information to support nursing practice, administration, education, and research; and to expand nursing knowledge. The purpose of nursing informatics is to: analyze information requirements; design, implement and evaluate information systems and data structures that support nursing; and identify and apply computer technologies for nursing."
- **Hannah, Ball & Edwards (1994):** "[U]se of information technologies in relation to those functions within the purview of nursing, and that are carried out by nurses when performing their duties. Therefore, any use of information technologies by nurses in relation to the care of their patients, the administration of healthcare facilities, or the educational preparation of individuals to practice the discipline is considered nursing informatics. For example, nursing informatics would include, but not be limited to, the use of artificial intelligence or decision-making systems to support the use of the nursing process; the use of a computer-based scheduling package to allocate staff in a hospital or healthcare organization; the

use of computers for patient education; the use of computer-assisted learning in nursing education; nursing use of a hospital information system; or research related to information nurses use in making patient care decisions and how those decisions are made." (p. 5)

- **American Nurses Association (1994):** "Nursing informatics is the specialty that integrates nursing science, computer science, and information science in identifying, collecting, processing, and managing data and information to support nursing practice, administration, education, research and the expansion of nursing knowledge." (p. 3)
- **Saba & McCormick (1995):** "It [nursing informatics] is concerned with the legitimate access to and use of data, information, and knowledge to standardize documentation, improve communication, and support decision-making process." (p. 222)
- **Saba & McCormick (1997):** "The use of technology and/or a computer system to collect, store, process, display, retrieve, and communicate timely data and information in and across healthcare facilities designed to administer nursing services and resources, manage delivery of patient and nursing care including documentation and planning, link research resources & findings to nursing practice, apply educational resources to nursing education, administer nursing services and resources, manage delivery of patient and nursing care including documentation and planning, link research resources & findings to nursing practice, and apply educational resources to nursing education."
- **Saba & McCormick (2001):** "Nursing informatics is a dynamic discipline, comprised of many aspects and defined in many ways. Definitions reflect the definer's perspectives and the emergence of new knowledge in nursing informatics and the sciences with which it is integrated."
- **Goossen (1996):** "Nursing informatics is the multi-disciplinary scientific endeavor of analyzing, formalizing and modeling how nurses collect and manage data, process data into information and knowledge, make knowledge-based decisions and inferences for patient care, and use this empirical and experiential knowledge in order to broaden the scope and enhance the quality of their professional practice."
- **International Medical Informatics Association—Nursing Informatics (IMIA-NI) (1998):** "Nursing informatics is the integration of nursing, its information, and information management with information processing and communication technology, to support the health of people worldwide."
- **Update 2010 from the Nursing Informatics Special Interest Group of the International Medical Informatics Association:** "Nursing informatics science and practice integrates nursing, its information and knowledge and their management with information and communication technologies to promote the health of people, families and communities worldwide."
- **Goossen (2000):** "Nursing informatics is the discipline that is concerned with the development, use, and evaluation of nursing information systems." (p. 25)
- **Goossen, W. T. F. (2000).** *Towards strategic use of nursing information in the Netherlands.* Amsterdam, Netherlands: Gegevens Koninklijke Bibliltheek Den Haag

- **ANA (2001):** "Nursing informatics is a specialty that integrates nursing science, computer science, and information science to manage and communicate data, information, and knowledge in nursing practice. Nursing informatics facilitates the integration of data, information, and knowledge to support patients, nurses, and other providers in their decision-making in all roles and settings. This support is accomplished through the use of information structures, information processes, and information technology." (p. 17)
- **Canadian Nurses Association (2001):** "Nursing Informatics (NI) is the application of computer science and information science to nursing. NI promotes the generation, management and processing of relevant data in order to use information and develop knowledge that supports nursing in all practice domains." (See http://www.cnia.ca/education.htm)
- **Canadian Nurses Association (2003):** "Nursing Informatics (NI): integrates nursing science, computer science, and information science to manage and communicate data, information, and knowledge in nursing practice. Nursing informatics facilitates the integration of data, information, and knowledge to support clients, nurses, and other providers in their decision-making in all roles and settings. This support is accomplished through the use of information structures, information processes, and information technology. The goal of nursing informatics is to improve the health of populations, communities, families, and individuals by optimizing information management and communication. This includes the use of information and technology in the direct provision of care, in establishing effective administrative systems, in managing and delivering educational experiences, in supporting lifelong learning, and in supporting nursing research." (See http://www.cnia.ca/education.htm)
- **Saba & McCormick (2006):** "The domain of nursing informatics is focused on data and its structures, information management, and the technology, including databases, needed to manage information effectively. Yet is also includes significant use of theory from linguistics, human-machine interface, decision science, cognitive science, communication, engineering, library science, and organizational dynamics." (see http://dlthede.net/informatics/chap01introni/ni_definitions.html)
- **Simpson (2006):** "Using technology, research, and professional experience to manage nursing data, information, and knowledge to improve practice and deliver better healthcare." (see http://dlthede.net/informatics/chap01introni/ni_definitions.html)
- **ANA (2008):** "Nursing informatics is a specialty that integrates nursing science, computer science, and information science to manage and communicate data, information, knowledge, and wisdom in nursing practice. Nursing informatics facilitates the integration of data, information, knowledge, and wisdom to support patients, nurses, and other providers in their decision-making in all roles and settings. This support is accomplished through the use of information structures, information processes, and information technology." (see http://dlthede.net/informatics/chap01introni/ni_definitions.html)

Despite all the aforementioned definitions, the focus of nursing informatics is on capturing data by using cognitive skills and managing the data, interpreted as information and converted to knowledge and wisdom for meaningful use in satisfactory care of the patients. Nursing informatics is focused on simplifying documentation with computer software and hardware technologies. With the help of nursing informatics, nurses' interactions with patients have altered the ways in which healthcare providers could diagnose, treat, and provide care for their patients.

HISTORY OF NURSING INFORMATICS

Historically, the field of nursing has encountered many milestones since the late 1800s, in which the world of technology has greatly acted as a catalyst toward the nursing informatics evolution. In the 21st century, technology has drastically revamped the United States healthcare delivery system (Tietze, 2012). Informatics deals with the gathering, storing, analyzing, transforming and relating of information gathered in a user-friendly format. In the United States, many healthcare organizations have information technology departments to handle the electronic flow of information. These departments play a crucial role in the decision-making process such as adoption of a new technology that will improve the delivery of care and efficiency. Some of the technologies such as electronic medical record (EMR) systems are responsible for the collection, transcription and storage of the patient's clinical data. Other systems include radiology and clinical laboratory record reporting systems; the pharmacy and nursing medication data reporting systems, which are responsible for the collection of pertinent information on medication monitoring to avoid errors, adverse reactions, and drug-drug/drug-food interaction; patients' scheduling for various healthcare procedures, including surgery suite and personnel material management; and financial systems for accurate billing and collections.

THE FUTURE IS HERE

The future of nursing informatics is centered on advances in accessing medical records, speed, development of new interactive software, information technology advancements such as image storage and transfer technology, and image technologies for storage of patient's medical records for easy accessibility. In addition, applications such as telehealth has made it possible for healthcare professionals to practice telemedicine from remote locations, and the move toward nanotechnology hand-held devices with biosensors that can be used for diagnosis and treatment are more cost effective than most expensive diagnosis equipment. New technologies are constantly shifting the practice of nursing, forecasting possibilities one cannot yet imagine, truly allowing the field of nursing to shift forward. With the new advances in technology and nursing practice as a whole, the definitions for nursing informatics are evolving, with constant revisions of both the definitions and scope of practice statements.

There is a great need for nurses to become computer literate. It is important to note that nursing does not only involve tasks, but also involves cognitive skills. Clinicians and nursing informatics are a joint function needed to support this process. Identifying and determining how to facilitate data collection is an informatics skill that all nurses need. Most of the nursing history and data have not been valued because they are either buried in paper patient records, which make retrieval an arduous task or worse impossible if the records are discarded when a patient is discharged. Paper documentation methods create other problems such as inconsistency and irregularity in charting, as well as lack of data evaluation and research.

Nursing informatics in today's nursing is critical. Nurses often spend a lot of time on documentation in addition to writing notes, but all these activities have been changed because, with nursing informatics, notes and charting can be recorded faster with a combination of computer software and hardware. Taking care of the patients is usually the focus of most nurses. Using technology to manage information in healthcare is known as informatics, hence the primary focus for nurses is information management, not computers. The nursing informatics role is to make the healthcare documentation user friendly and easy for documentation and elimination of the amount of time spent in gathering information from the patient's chart.

INFORMATICS TOOLS

Nursing informatics can help nurses and other healthcare providers with the implementation of various technological systems such as barcode systems, computerized physician order entry (CPOE), and portable computers. The Leapfrog Group and the Veterans Administration's National Center for Patient Safety created an initiative with the Bar-Code Medication Administration system to improve the accuracy of patient identification. Before the nurse administers medication, especially to a high-risk patient, the nurse would match the barcode found on the unit-dose medication package with the patient identification bracelet. The barcode system emphasizes the six rights of drug administration; it allows for the correct allocation of the medication to the right client, thus preventing human error. The scanner will show a list of medications and the times of administration. Other features of the bar code scanner are automatic documentation and the reduction of adverse effects. The machine warns healthcare providers of possible allergies and adverse drug interaction. For example, a client who is allergic to penicillin could greatly reduce the adverse effects with this information imported into the barcode system. If another nurse orders a variant of penicillin, the tool will alert the nurse, preventing an error from occurring. Therefore, the workload of the nurse will drastically decrease; he or she will not have to sort through endless paperwork or medication cards for the client, which has become outdated. Also, this allows for information to be accessed in a timely manner and will not permit time to be wasted with relaying information from nurse to nurse. The decreased amount of time spent with medication administration and documentation will increase quality patient care. As stated best by Manno, this technological advancement, "will make it easy to do the right thing and hard to do the wrong thing" (as cited in Czar & Hebda, 2009).

Another tool that has advanced the healthcare field is the computerized physician order entry (CPOE). This is a computerized documentation system in which physicians, nurse practitioners, or other healthcare providers enter orders into an information system.

This system will shrink documentation errors while creating a more accurate order when compared to handwritten documentation. It acts as an alarm system, notifying the healthcare provider when critical lab values are needed or certain tests are due. It also allows for the different healthcare entities such as the hospitals, pharmacy, and laboratory systems to interact and communicate, allowing for a faster, more effective and efficient healthcare system. Each entity is notified of potential adverse effects of medications, dosage problems, contradictions, etc. This system allows for the processing and management of data (i.e., lab values) to be interpreted into information, synthesized into knowledge, and identified as problems, leading to further medical intervention. The transformation of processing and managing data to the recognition of identifying problems for medical intervention is "the key concept of nursing informatics" (Tietze, 2012). This automation is the reference database, which will allow for nurses to retrieve and review updated information on medications.

The portable computer, also known as the peanut, is another tool that has advanced the nursing profession with respect to technology. This portable hand-held computer manufactured by the National Cash Register (NCR) company has generated lots of interest among nursing professionals. The peanut has ample memory, which allows for the nurse to input vital signs and other pertinent data at a patient's bedside. The peanut will display chart and medical records right at the time of administration. This portable device is extremely accessible because it prevents the nurse from traveling to the nursing station for documentation. This simple yet brilliant device will allow for the nurse to spend more time with each client, creating a better nursing-client relationship, which, therefore, will improve client care. From a personal standpoint, the peanut has allowed less medical errors and more accurate and up-to-date client information, as well as making the assessment and diagnosis quick and efficient (Pocklington, Rieder, & Saba, 1989).

COMPETENT NURSE EQUATES LESS STRESS WITH DECREASED WORK LOAD

With the new technological shift of the healthcare industry, patient care has improved exponentially, creating a healthier patient and a more competent nurse due to less stress with a decreased work load. For example, upon arrival, a client entering the emergency department, in which the nurse notices the client is experiencing shortness of breath and chest pain, a narration from this scenario may involve performing a physical assessment of the client, which entails taking vital signs with specific episodic assessment. Today, vital signs are recorded using monitoring devices; this allows the nurse to work effectively and faster. First, the objective data would be collected from the vital signs and the patient's interview. Next, the client's past medical history could possibly be viewed through computerized-archived patient data, in which it will be organized and interpreted into information. Finally, if the dropping of the respiration rate is abnormal, then quick medical treatment is needed. The transitions of the vital signs (data) to knowledge (the awareness of the abnormal respiration rate) are the key components of nursing informatics. In retrospect, in this case study the client complains of chest pain. An immediate diagnostic test can be checked with a medical tech device such as an electrocardiogram, also known as an ECG. The nurse will attach electrodes to the skin of the client, which records the electrical activity of the heart. If there was an abnormality in the heart muscle, it would not contract fully, leading to a sign of a dysthymia. The use of technology, ECG allows the nurse to make a nursing diagnosis (clinical judgment) in a timely and effective manner, therefore allowing the need to implement a plan of care for the client's well-being. These quality measures intertwine technology with the dynamic and cyclic process of the nursing process.

INFORMATICS AND RESEARCH

Furthermore, evidenced-based research via data mining is a new research method that is fast evolving, especially with the mandated adoption of electronic health records in 2014. Many hospitals are taking advantage of this research methodology for their pilot studies prior to the bench work and grant applications. Hospital registries are being utilized for data extraction, patterning, analyses, and sharing with the help of biostatisticians and bio-informaticist. Personally, the author, Okunji (2010) and the dissertation team foresaw this future research innovation and took advantage of it in 2006 when they utilized the HCUP NIS large population database in the study of the "Effects of Patients and Hospital Characteristics on Inpatients with Diabetic Myocardial Infarction."

In summary, technology has radically transformed the healthcare industry especially in providing sufficient care for each client. New developments in other areas, such as in distance teaching and evidenced-based research, will drastically affect the role of healthcare professionals, academia, and researchers. Also, the specialty of nursing informatics will soon become a leading contender in the job market and it will truly revamp the healthcare system as we know it today. An editorial in *Nursing Forum* gives a philosophical overview by asking, "What will automation mean for nursing and nurses?" and pleading with nurses not to adopt nursing's historic weapon against change, passive resistance, which could lead us to professional suicide, but to think positively and plan now for the automated world in which we are destined to live.

COMPUTER AND INFORMATION LITERACY

There is a great need for nurses to be computer and information literate in today's healthcare environment. In 2004, President Bush called for adoption of interoperable electronic records for most Americans by the year 2014. Healthcare is in transition and nursing is affected by these changes. The use of technology is mandatory and a background in computer and nursing is necessary because nursing informatics is an integral part of nursing. The old way of patient care is gone; today, with several specialties, consults, medications, laboratory reports, and procedures, the paper system is inadequate. A well-designed information system developed based on nursing needs will facilitate finding and using information for patient care. Information skills enable nurses to participate in and benefit from this process. To improve healthcare, it is imperative to have a workforce that can innovate and implement information technology. Ultimately, nurses have a major role to play in informatics. Nursing informatics is designed to improve nursing documentation, which can be used to expand knowledge, which in turn translates to quality healthcare. From nursing documentation, one can easily see the relationship between nursing diagnoses, interventions, and outcomes for patients. Without knowledge of the chain of events, the only thing left is intuition and old knowledge to use when making decisions about the best interventions in patient care. Informatics can furnish the information needed to see these relationships and to provide care based on actual patient data.

INFORMATICS AND NURSING EDUCATION

Furthermore, informatics is being used in distance teaching and learning in most institutions. Online education has become the wave of the future in which busy and professional individuals may now earn their degrees without leaving the comfort of their homes, leaving work or neglecting to take care of their families. Many nursing institutions are now implementing RN-to-BSN programs for the associate RNs as more and more states are now mandating that by 2020 the baccalaureate level would be the required degree to be employed in acute care institutions. Furthermore, it has been proven that there is a high correlation between higher education in nursing and positive outcomes on discharge. An already existing institutional system such as Blackboard could be used to plan, develop, implement, and evaluate online or hybrid teaching and learning tracks by a nurse informatics specialist (Okunji & Hill, 2013).

TABLE 4.1 Nursing Informatics contribution to the *Undergraduate* Program AACN Standards by Outcomes: Dr. Okunji's Course Evaluation

AACN STANDARDS	OUTCOMES
Synthesize knowledge from liberal arts, sciences, humanities, and nursing disciplines in critical thinking and decision making for the implementation, management, and evaluation of safe, holistic care for individuals, families, and communities.	Nursing informatics is instilled to the students on how data could be transformed to information, then into knowledge that enables informed judgment (critical thinking) that gives the safe care that patients receive.
Practice professional nursing within ethical, legal, and professional standards of practice.	Students understand the concept of HIPAA as it relates to all e-patients' information.
Provide culturally competent care across the life span in partnership with the inter-professional healthcare team.	Provides students with information confidentiality, privacy, and security across the life span.
Demonstrate communication skills essential to the role of the nurse as provider, designer, manager, coordinator of care, and member of the profession.	Students learn the relevance of timely information in patient safety.

TABLE 4.1 Nursing Informatics contribution to the *Undergraduate* Program AACN Standards by Outcomes: Dr. Okunji's Course Evaluation (*Continued*)

AACN STANDARDS	OUTCOMES
Collaborate with colleagues and other members of the inter-professional health team to promote health and well-being to individuals, families, and communities.	SimChart® used to simulate EHR systems that all healthcare professionals must input for holistic care from admission to discharge with families and community collaboration.
Engage in professional role behaviors that serve to improve nursing and healthcare delivery systems and address the changing needs of a multicultural society.	Students understand that professional integrity that involves in information transfer is critical to patient safety.
Apply leadership and management skills to provide quality, cost-effective nursing in a variety of settings.	Students understand that the use of informatics systems results in quality care and is cost effective.
Engage in critical inquiry and incorporate evidence-based research in the practice of professional nursing.	The discussion board exposes the students to thought-provoking questions and discussions that lead to a good outcome.

Source: Okunji (2012), Unpublished Nurse Informatics Course Evaluation Form.

References

American Nurses Association. (1994). *The scope of practice for nursing informatics*. Washington, DC: Author.

American Nurses Association. (2001). *Scope and standards of nursing informatics practice*. Washington, DC: Author.

American Nurses Association (2008). *Nursing informatics: Scope and standards of practice*. Washington, DC: Author.

American Nurses Association Council on Computers in Nursing. (1995). Report on the designation of nursing informatics as a specialty. Congress of Nursing Practice unpublished report. In Saba, V., & McCormick, K. (Eds.), *Essentials of computers for nursing*. (2nd ed.). New York, NY: McGraw-Hill.

Canadian Nurses Association. (2001). Nursing Informatics Definitions over the past 30 years. http://dlthede.net/informatics/chapo1introni/ni_definitions.html

Canadian Nurses Association. (2003). Nursing Informatics Definition over the past 30 years. http://dlthede.net/informatics/chapo1introni/ni_definitions.html

Collen, M. (1995). *A history of medical informatics in the United States, 1950 to 1990*. Indianapolis, IN: American Medical Informatics Association.

Czar, P., & Hebda, T., (2009). *Handbooks of informatics for nurses & healthcare professionals*. Upper Saddle River, NJ: Pearson.

Graves, J. R., & Corcoran, S. (1989). The study of nursing informatics. *Image: The Journal of Nursing Scholarship, 21*(4), 227–231.

Goossen, W. T. F. (1996). Nursing information management and processing: A framework and definition for systems analysis, design and evaluation. *International Journal of Biomedical*

Computing, 40(3), 187–195.

Goossen, W. T. F. (2000). *Towards strategic use of nursing information in the Netherlands*. Amsterdam, Netherlands: Gegevens Koninklijke Biblitheek Den Haag.

Hannah, K. J. & Ball, M. J. & Edwards, K. J. (1999). *Introduction to nursing informatics* (2nd ed.). New York, NY: Springer.

Hannah, K. (1985). Current trends in nursing informatics: Implications for curriculum planning. In K. J. Hannah, E. J. Guillemin & D. K. Conklin (Eds.), *Nursing uses of computers and information science: Proceedings of the IFIP=IMIA international symposium on nursing uses of computers and information science* (pp. 181–187). Amsterdam, Netherlands: Elsevier.

International Medical Informatics Association. (1998). *Nursing Informatics Definitions over the past 30 years*. http://dlthede.net/informatics/chapo1introni/ni_definitions.html

McGonigle, E. & Eggers, R. (1991). Establishing a nursing informatics program. *Computers in Nursing 9*(5), 174–179.

Okunji, P. O., (2010). Outcomes of patients with diabetic myocardial infarction in non-federal hospitals: Effects of hospital and patient characteristics (Dissertation). *ProQuest® Dissertation Database*, AAT 3442071

Okunji P. O., & Hill, M (2013). Undergraduate online program development, Implementation and evaluation: A pilot study. *Canadian Journal of Nursing Informatics, 8*(3–4), 1–9.

Saba, V. K. & McCormick, K. A. (1995). *Essentials of computers for nurses* (2nd ed.). New York, NY: McGraw Hill.

Saba, V. K. & McCormick, K. (1997, July 21). A National Informatics Agenda for Nursing Education and Practice. *Report to the Secretary of the Department of Health & Human Services*. Rockville, Maryland.

Saba, V. K. & McCormick, K. A. (2001). *Essentials of computers for nurses* (3rd ed.). New York, NY: McGraw Hill.

Sackett, K. M. & Erdley, W. S. (2002). The history of health care informatics. In S. Englebardt, & R. Nelson (Eds.), *Health care informatics: An interdisciplinary approach* (pp. 453–477). St. Louis, MO: Mosby.

Saba, V. K. & McCormick, K. A. (2001). *Essentials of computers for nurses* (4th ed). New York: McGraw Hill, p. 184.

Scholes, M. & Barber, B. (1980). Towards nursing informatics. In D. A. D. Lindberg & S. Kaihara (Eds.), *MEDINFO: 1980* (pp. 7–73). Amsterdam, Netherlands: North-Holland.

Simpson, R. (2006). Coherent heterogeneity: Redefining nursing in a consumer-smart world. In H. A. Park, P. Murray, & C. Delaney, C. (Eds.), *Consumer-centered computer-supported care for healthy people*. Amsterdam, Netherlands: IOS Press.

Saba, V., Rieder, K. A., Pocklington, D. B. (1989) *Nursing and computers: An anthology*. New York, NY: Springer. 10.1007/978-1-4612-3622-1

Tietze, M. (2012). Nursing informatics: What's it all about? *Continuing Education*. Retrieved from www.uta.edu/ced/static/onlinecne/CEAugust08.pdf

CHAPTER 5

External Drivers of Informatics Technology

CHAPTER HIGHLIGHTS

This chapter discusses the following:

- How factors outside of the organization will not only influence, but drive the use of informatics technology within any organization
- How cost containment is the key driving force of informatics outside of healthcare and financing of the healthcare delivery systems in the United States
- How Informatics, medical, and nursing technologies in the United States have global impact in terms of cost commitment and cost control by other nations
- How the United States, and across the globe, incorporation of a cost-effectiveness analysis with sound informatics processes in the healthcare delivery systems is appropriate and the right thing to do

THERE ARE FACTORS outside of organizations that will not only influence, but drive the use of informatics technology. Since the later part of the 20th century, the United States and other developed nations have been experiencing tremendous technological shifts in the delivery of healthcare systems due to increase in technological innovations such as information technology. These forces continue to alter the trends and directions in healthcare delivery systems in the United States, as in illness to wellness, acute care to primary care, inpatient to outpatient, individual health to community health and well-being, fragmented care to managed care, independent institutions to integrated systems, service duplication to continuum of services, and the demand for latest medical innovation by consumers who are more knowledgeable and have more access to information via the cyber space than ever before.

HEALTHCARE COST CONTAINMENT

The primary reasons for the aforementioned trends are the promotion of healthcare at the least cost and the change in the concept of health itself. The concept of health is now changing to wellness (Akaho et al., 1998). Some of the forces outside of the system that continue to shape the healthcare delivery system are the political climate of the country, economic development, technological progress, and cultural and social values (e.g., ethnic and cultural diversities, Congress, interest groups, laws and regulations and the population characteristic, such as the demographic and health trends and the global influences). Lastly, the Patient Protection and Affordable Care Act (ACA) of 2010, popularly known as Obama Care, which promises to reduce the uninsured by 32 million people, (Henry J. Kaiser Family Foundation, 2011) has been the best so far for the underinsured and uninsured population, especially for those with preexisting conditions. Although this act may be reversed due to high unexpected cost increase on evaluation of the act, it would be appropriate for an option to be in place before its replacement or at least to amend a portion of the act, rather than creating a total replacement.

The key driving force of informatics outside of healthcare is the cost containment and financing of the healthcare delivery systems in the United States. New technology comes with enormous price. It is well known that most sophisticated diagnostic tests have resulted in the reduction of complications and disability and has reduced hospital length of stay (LOS). Similarly, new medications and medical cures have increased longevity of life and have added good and/or better quality of life with the stability of chronic illness, especially in the elderly and disable citizens. To keep up with the influx of technology, research is necessary. Research typically is very costly and can take years to develop, thereby increasing the cost of new knowledge. There will also be a need for more skilled and well-trained staff to put this technology into practice. This is an added expense to the organization. Well-educated consumers who have access to information (via the Internet), demand new technology as soon as it is available irrespective of the cost, especially if insurance or the government is covering the cost. The need for cost containment continues to drive the use of informatics with the healthcare delivery system.

GLOBAL IMPLICATIONS

Informatics, medical, and nursing technologies in the United States have global impact in terms of cost commitment and cost control by other nations. The rest of the world tends to wait for new technological innovations from American companies; the technologies are replicated and then introduced into other countries' healthcare delivery systems without the initial cost burdens. If there is a slow pace in informatics and technological developments in the United States, there may be serious health consequences in the global communities. Informatics and telemedicine had made online education, medical, and nursing research possible in areas where these phenomena may not have been possible worldwide (Umar, 2003).

Despite the global accessibility to technology and informatics, global communities are faced with the impacts on bioethics and costs. With this convenience comes responsibility and accountability for healthcare professionals and organizations that utilize the new technologies and informatics. Increasing incidents of ethical and moral issues come up more frequently due to informatics and advanced technological techniques in healthcare and other fields. As Sewell and Thede (2013) rightly pointed out,

> The application of Informatics and Information technology has become indispensable in the delivery of efficient and cost effective management of health care in this modern age, not only in the United States but globally. With the growth of the internet applications, the e-health [industry] is fast becoming

a growing field within the healthcare industry. Currently, Telemedicine and Telehealth technologies are used in both synchronous and asynchronous applications to deliver medical care when the healthcare provider and the recipient of care are separated by distance. (Sewell & Thede, 2013)

All these aforementioned advances are costly to the healthcare industry and many times to the patients who may be paying out of pocket. The United States remains at the forefront in the new age of technology and informatics. The uncontrolled use of medical technology and informatics continues to cause a very deep concern about the ever-rising costs of medical care.

CHALLENGES: COST EFFECTIVENESS AND RISKS

Another healthcare cost challenge is that the average American healthcare consumer always wants all the available medical resources and technology used whenever there is a need to promote health and/or life with regards to how small the benefit will be in relation to the costs. Physicians and advanced practice nurses always find themselves in very difficult situations when the insurance companies require that treatments be withheld because of cost inefficiency. Both the healthcare consumers and the American public frown at this phenomenon whenever and where ever they happen. Even the members of Congress and law makers are also concerned when cost effectiveness is brought into the picture of the healthcare delivery systems in the United States. Yet, the law makers are reluctant to fund health research through the National Institute of Health due to costs. However, more expensive care may be more cost effective when used appropriately (e.g., CAT scans are more expensive than X-ray imaging. However, CAT scans can reduce surgical needs) (Nitzkin, 1996).

It becomes very important for the United States and countries across the globe to incorporate a cost-effective analysis with sound informatics processes in the healthcare delivery systems as appropriate. The cost-effective analysis incorporates costs and benefits, especially those benefits that cannot be quantified in dollars and cents. Whenever the cost cannot be expressed in monetary terms, it may be expressed in terms of the number of service units, space requirements, staff times, the degree of specialization required to provide the care, years of lives saved by the treatments, hospitalization and early return to work, quality of life, and quality of life. All these points will drive the informatics processes.

Risk is another nonmonetary cost associated with any procedure. No medical procedure is completely safe and without risk, even if it is only the risk of infection due to surgery and loss of skin integrity. Sometimes the risks associated with healthcare procedures may be minimal and at times very significant with undesirable side effects, medical complications, injuries to the patient, or even death. The monetary measures of these unfortunate incidents can be very difficult to estimate because the cost-and-risk benefit evaluations are not precise or objective. Each one is subjective and based on professional opinion and/or judgment. In any case, informatics and standardization of clinical guidelines based on evidence-based practice will be more objective.

In conclusion, technology and informatics have impacted and positively influenced the delivery of healthcare delivery systems in the United States and globally. Additionally, they have both influenced and enhanced quality of life. At this point, many healthcare organizations, small and/or large, cannot operate efficiently without computer-based information systems. The United States remains the leader in the technological world. However, most of these technologies are borrowed or purchased by developing or third-world countries. Hence, the healthcare supplies and equipment developments with current policies on traded tariffs in the United States have critical implications on global health, with ethical and moral concerns. All these concerns continue to drive the use of informatics in healthcare settings and other areas of disciplines.

References

Akaho, E. et al. (1998). A proposed optimal health care system based on a comprehensive study conducted between Canada and Japan. *Canadian Journal of Public Health, 89*(5), 301–307.

Fuchs, V. R. (2004). More variation in use of care, more flat-to-the-curve medicine. *Health Affairs, 23*, 104–107.

Henry J. Kaiser Family Foundation (2011). *Summary of coverage provisions in the Patient Protection and Affordable Care Act.* Retrieved from https://www.kff.org/health-costs/issue-brief/summary-of-coverage-provisions-in-the-patient/

Nitzkin, J. L. (1996). Technology and health care—Driving costs up, not down. *IEEE Technology and Social Magazine, 15*(3), 40–45.

Sewell, J. P., & Thede, L. Q. (2013). Medical terminology. Retrieved from http://samples.jbpub.com/9781284035452/Chapter5.pdf

Umar, K., (2003). Telemedicine works: Quality, access, and cost impacts cited. Closing the gap. Washington, DC: Department of Health and Human Services.

CHAPTER 6

Nurse Executives and the Use of Informatics in Documentation and Other Administrative Activities

CHAPTER HIGHLIGHTS

This chapter discusses the following:

- How nurse administrators are using informatics to rise above the basics and extend their clinical information system skills to areas of financial management, process improvement, benchmarking, and business intelligence
- How informatics could assist nurse administrators to use data to demonstrate correlative relationships in their clinical practice area such as staffing and the possible positive financial outcome as a result of appropriate staffing levels
- How forecasting can also be determined by comparisons of falls, pressure ulcers, infections, call bell response time, management in patients' pain, patient satisfaction, and a host of other variables

NURSE EXECUTIVES AND COMPUTER APPLICATIONS

IT IS OBVIOUS that nurse managers and administrators must have a vast array of knowledge, competency, and technical skills to be most effective in their roles. Information management and technology fall under one of the five leadership domains defined by the American Organization of Nurse Executives (AONE, 2013). The amount of both information and data is growing exponentially, and the technology to provide information is rapidly and constantly changing. Due to these changes, chief nurse executives (CNE) are in a strategic role for healthcare systems. It is essential that an administrator has the basic competencies and beyond in information management (Mays, Wanda, & Kathleen, 2008). Nurse administrators are expected to rise above the basics and extend their clinical information system skills to areas of financial management, process improvement, benchmarking, and business intelligence.

This chapter will explore the administration (nurse managers, nurse executives, nurse administrators) tools necessary for role efficiency. It will identify the tools necessary to manage business processes in nursing services, demonstrate basic competencies in spreadsheets and flowcharting in nursing administration, and discuss data management to improve outcomes using quality improvement, benchmarking, and patient care. It will also explore the use of specialized applications in nursing administration, including scheduling systems and patient classification systems.

BUDGETS AND VARIANCE REPORTS

The AONE has published guiding principles in information management and technology that describe the responsibility of nurse executives. These guidelines include the use of various tools, such as computer applications. Spreadsheets are useful tool to any nurse manager to monitor monthly budgets, create variance reports, and establish if a relationship exists between two groups of data. Important data can easily be misinterpreted or relationships in that data can be missed altogether if viewed independently.

FORECASTING

Evidence-based knowledge is a critical move for leadership in any organization today. Hence, making numbers talk is the new way of doing things in today's healthcare arena. Mays, Wanda, and Kathleen (2008) iterated that "perhaps the most essential information competency for nurse executives is the ability to discern data from information or to take raw data and make it into information" (Mays et al., 2008). Nurse administrators can use data to demonstrate correlative relationships in their clinical practice area, such as staffing, and the possible positive financial outcome as a result of appropriate staffing levels. Comparisons of falls, pressure ulcers, infections, call bell response time, management in patients' pain, and patient satisfaction could also be made. Although healthcare and its demands on nurses can be unpredictable, data can be formulated into spreadsheets to assist in interpreting historical data, graphing trends and seasonal patterns and predicting future needs. It has been stated by some researchers that effective forecasting needs to encompass 1–5 years of data (Sewell & Thede, 2013). Capture of data over too short of a period can lead to drawing false conclusions. It is then not truly reflective of the actual trends.

OUTCOMES SYSTEMS

The nurse administrator has the responsibility for improving clinical outcomes of the organization. Process or performance improvement requires the identification, analysis, and improvement of processes already in place to meet quality, safety, customer satisfaction and financial goals. Hence, "the CNE uses clinical performance improvement goals as an integration strategy to align disparate and often conflicting priorities in the organization" (Englebright & Perlin, 2008). There are multiple strategies that can be used by administrators to initiate and implement process improvements. The key is an organized approach to plan for needed changes. Tools such as spreadsheets, flow charts, and cause-and-effect charts can provide a visual aid in this highly analytical process. Flowcharts are very useful and serve as a visual aid to making processes more efficient or to eliminate variations in processes. They allow for identification of unnecessary steps that can be eliminated to yield a more seamless flow. Relationships among complex processes can be more easily examined through cause-and-effect charting, or fishbone charting. It places the effect at one end of the chart and then all the suspected variables that may be the cause are branched off. These diagrams can be readily and sufficiently created through simple software packages already on hand and used in Microsoft Word.

SYSTEMS INTEROPERABILITY

It is also the responsibility of the nurse administrator to take charge of the planning, implementation, and evaluation of several and sometimes complex projects. These projects could have financial implications and involve numerous organizational key stakeholders. Although not typically used by nurse administrators, there are project management software programs designed to assist in providing needed organization to keep projects on time and within their allotted budget. It gives the opportunity to track the projects' progress. These programs can demonstrate start/stop dates, milestones, and costs as they relate to specific tasks and timeline/deadlines of tasks to be completed. It may also have a linking feature that can update the entire project when there is a change on one end of the project. E-mails can also be automatically generated and sent as a reminder to upcoming dates and deadlines. This will give the administrator more time to focus on the bigger issue at hand, the project. Reports can also be generated and provide project cost analysis. There are many project management software programs available on the market. Purchasers of these programs must consider the interoperability of these systems with other administrative tools. The number of users to access the program, the security of the program, and the overall cost of purchasing and implementation must also be considered. If this is to be a frequently utilized resource, then it may be well worth the institution's financial investment.

HUMAN RESOURCE SYSTEMS

Nurse administrators must also become quite familiar with human resource management systems (HRMS). These systems are vital in appropriately planning for staffing of nursing services. Personnel, staffing, and employment information can be effectively managed by HRMS. It manages personnel files, work schedules and requests, payroll, licensure, education, and skill qualifications. This system also proves to be critical in aggregating nursing and patient care data for nurse managers to track, trend, and analyze productivity for benchmarking within their organizations. Common minimum requirements that an HRMS system need to contain are handling scheduling for 24 hours a day, 7 days per week, accommodate different scheduling rules for units across an entire organization or network, allow for staff scheduling, determine the right number and mix of nursing staff for patient needs, provide an analysis of nursing staff usage to manage productivity and support quality patient outcomes, track time and attendance, connect to the payroll system, retain certification and licensure information, and serve as a repository for competency assessment and annual employee appraisals (Sewell & Thede, 2013).

BENCHMARKING

In previous years, nursing and their services had always been perceived as an added hospital expense. This was mostly because revenue was generated by hospital admissions and by the care provided. As we all know, that was the old way. With the advent of the Affordable Care Act associated with healthcare reform, the focus is now on the quality of patient care provided. Reimbursements will be gauged on benchmarking and performance.

Benchmarking is defined "as a process of continuous measuring and comparing an organization's business against others and is one of the approaches to obtain useful data results, and reporting performances are thought to be key strategies for influencing market forces, and evidence supports positive effects of performance reporting" (De Korne et al., 2012, pp. 187–198). According to George, Shelly, Cynthia, Naomi, and Claire (2013), "Public reporting of relevant data enables healthcare consumers to contribute and make critically informed decisions about the healthcare with their primary care providers" (pp. 68–75). Nurses are at the core of this initiative to improve quality, improve patient satisfaction, and prevent healthcare errors. Therefore, it is imperative that nurse administrators must remain keen and in tune with progress of improvements to foster a culture of excellence in patient care among their staff. Not only are these administrators involved in hospital base performance initiatives, but they are also held to those mandated by the Center for Medicare and Medicaid (CMS). These mandated programs include Consumer Assessment of Health Providers, Hospital Survey (HCAHPS) and core measures. Administrators can also affiliate themselves with the national database of nursing quality indicators (NDNQI). This organization requires administration to appoint staff and resources in the collection, aggregation, submission of data, and response to reports.

QUALITY CONTROL

Standardized core measures are required by all accredited healthcare organizations through the Hospital Inpatient Quality Reporting program. These measures were first established by the Joint Commission (TJC), the CMS, and the Hospital Quality Alliance (HQA) in 1998. Core measures have grown in health disparities captured since their inception. They currently review myocardial infarction, pneumonia, congestive heart failure, treatment of asthma in children, pregnancy, and surgical care. To stay compliant with extensive data collection, aggregation and reporting is required. Hence George and colleagues (2013) comment that "these data are made available through www.hospitalcompare.hhs.gov and the method of transparency further emphasizes the need for highly reliable data abstraction practices" (pp. 68–75).

STANDARDIZATION

Due to the increasing demand on healthcare facilities for quality care, the CMS, in conjunction with the HQA, now require hospitals to survey patients and their families in regards to their healthcare experience. The standardized survey tool, known as the Hospital Consumer Assessment of Healthcare Providers and Systems (HCAHPS), is administered to a random selection of discharged patients. It was designed by the Agency for Healthcare Research and Quality. This information is submitted for trending and benchmarking through the CMS website. This provides another means of public accountability in healthcare. The process of surveying patients can be outsourced to a private company or can be performed with hospital employees. Either way, there is a standardized method of data collection using a set of 18 questions formulated by the CMS. Institutions can customize this tool by adding their own questions.

QUALITY MEASURES

Consumer Assessment of Health Providers, Hospital Survey (HCAHPS) measure the patient experience and some areas of core measures. These factors are influenced by the quality of nursing care received. The safety and quality initiative for nurses is the National Database of Nursing Quality Indicators® (NDNQI®), which delivers evidence to support the importance of nurse-sensitive measures in overall patient experience strategy that nurse administrators can voluntarily participate in. The NDNQI® is a national database to which hospitals submit sensitive nursing data about structure, process, and outcomes of nursing care (Sewell & Thede, 2013). This data is then compiled quarterly and reported to participant hospitals. The data reported includes but is not limited to intravenous infiltration, falls, restraint use, nursing turn over, pressure ulcers, nursing hours per patient day, staff mix, infections, and nosocomial infections. Additional information regarding the NDNQI initiative can be found at www.nursingquality.org.

MANAGEMENT SOFTWARE

There are multiple data elements collected in regards to patient care delivery by nursing services every day. Nurse administrators must be diligent enough to differentiate and focus on a few elements that pertain to their specific clinical area that will produce effective, quality care. Nurse administrators need to also use a sense of business intelligence in which they would ensure that they align their specific unit elements with that of the organizational goals. In collaboration with information management specialists and hospital leadership, nurse administrators need to develop a strategic plan for business intelligence. Information systems management can assist in the development or selection of data warehousing software, dashboard software, data integration software, and querying software to communicate performance indicators. This process requires an integrated approach from all departments and all levels of administration. Dashboards allow for real-time deliverance of performance indicators such as staffing, productivity, costs, and quality. The need of these devices has a greater need today than ever before. It is necessary for anyone who has decision-making responsibility to have access to information in an expeditious manner.

The throughput process, also known as clinical workflow, continues to be a challenge to acute care hospitals today. All various types of delays in patient care in the hospital setting ultimately affect the profitability of the institution. There are systems now available on the market that can reduce the delays and innovate the delivery of healthcare. McKesson and CareLogistics are two examples of these systems. Compared to dashboards, these patient care management systems provide an improvement of patient care by keeping managers informed in real time through synchronization of patient rooms, tasks, services, equipment, and patient locations, with alerts for priority.

SCHEDULING SYSTEMS

Some institutions continue to schedule nursing staff by using a paper system. Computerized employee scheduling systems have many benefits to be considered. The time managers spend completing the repetitive tasks of staff scheduling, taking into consideration scheduling rules, master schedules, shift rotations, and requests for time off, these systems can handle all these scheduling variations, making the first draft of a schedule much timelier. Nurse availability is shown in the system and modifications can be made more easily around them. It can also serve as a protective measure to prevent mis-scheduling of staff. It can also generate reports that are necessary to demonstrate education hours, leave hours, vacation hours, and number of productive hours in a pay period. This information or selected information can be shared with staff through the intranet or e-mail and allow nursing staff to be interactive with their schedules as well. Some software applications, such as *Bid for Health*, allow nurses that meet the qualifications of an open shift need to place a bid for that shift while being offered an incentive. This method of staffing has been reported by Sewell & Thede (2013) to reduce the costs of labor contracting by several million dollars per year and has increased nurses staffing satisfaction because of the autonomy in self-scheduling.

STAFF MANAGEMENT

With the knowledge that staffing is a difficult daily management, task-patient classification systems were created to assist leaders in making this task a more prudent decision-making process. It allows for consideration of patient acuity, time-base activities, nursing diagnoses, treatments, medications, and activities of daily living in relation to the full-time equivalents needed for a nursing unit. All these systems are dependent on timely and accurate entry of patient acuity and other related data. Some systems require manual input of this information, while others automatically pull this data from the electronic medical record, alleviating the extra step. It is vital that a nurse's documentation is current to give an up-to-date and accurate acuity representation.

DOCUMENTATION SYSTEMS

As healthcare in America continues to drive toward a complete electronic record system within hospitals, it has been reported by Sewell & Thede (2013) that this is actually the case in less than 1% of U.S. hospitals and only 50% have clinical documentation systems. Nurse administrators will also be faced with the challenge of the selection, purchase, and integration of a clinical information system or a module to correspond with the system. Nurse administrators need to possess an intricate understanding of the capabilities and limitations of such systems to be an effective voice for nursing. They would act as advocates for all of nursing and the improvement of the nursing care process. Although nurse administrators delegate portions of the clinical information system implementation process, according to a statement by the American Organization of Nurse Executives, the administrator holds the accountability for the process (Sewell & Thede, 2013). This accountability includes development of a strategic plan, knowing about the planned technology and its implications on nursing services, understanding the legal implications in regards to data ownership, visiting other institutions where the potential system has been implemented, preparing for the impact of the training process, developing a timeline for implementation and adhering to it, include health science schools affiliated with the institution and those who utilize the facility to lessen their strain, making preparations for system down times. Government-mandated implementation of electronic health records (EHR) started in 2011 and as of 2014 institutions who failed to meet meaningful use requirements of EHR had reduction in Medicare reimbursements. The Association of Nurse Executives also give suggestions on how the nurse administrators need to handle the meaningful use legislation: strategize about implementation with attention to clinical workflow implications, be aware of phase-in regulations so that reimbursements are not affected, and assure that vendor products are certified (American Organization of Nurse Executives [AONE], 2013).

CLINICAL TOOLS

It is essential for nurse administrators to understand and use computer application programs in their daily duties, as with all other health professionals. With their role in the monitoring, trending, and reporting of mandated, benchmarked quality improvement data to government agencies, this continues to prove to be vital. Nurse administrators will continue to have a great need for access to the tools necessary to improve patient care, meet regulatory requirements, and support financial decision matters. However, "the best tools will not be developed without nursing leaders taking the initiative to describe what information they need and how they need it to be designed and executives are the best advocates for the development of decision support systems that provide quality safety, and financial data in a format easily used for making correlations" (Mays, 2008). These system tools, scheduling, human resource management, patient flow management, and acuity management, all support effective and efficient administrative work. It is important not to forget the power of the administrator's voice in the advocacy in the purchase of information systems and to remain an authoritative, responsible, and accountable role in obtaining and providing the necessary resources to accomplish patient care in a safe and effective manner.

References

American Organization of Nurse Executives (2013). AONE 2013 Year End Report. Retrieved from http://www.aone.org/docs/2013-year-end-report.pdf

De korne, D., Van Wijngaarden, J., Sol, K., Betz, R., Thomas, R., Schein, O., & Klazinga, N. (2012). Hospital benchmarking: Are U.S. eye hospitals ready? *Health Care Management Review, 37*(2), 187–198. http://dx.doi.org/10.1097/HMR.0b013e31822aa46d

Englebright, J., & Perlin, J. (2008). The chief nurse executive role in large healthcare systems. *Nursing Administration Quarterly, 32*(3), 188–194.

George, H., Davis, S., Mitchell, C., Moyer, N., & Toner, C. (2013). Abstraction of core measure data: Creating a process for interrater reliability. *Nursing Care Quality, 28*(1), 68–75.

Mays, C., Wanda K., & Kathleen S. (2008). Keeping up, the nurse executive's present and future role in information technology. *Nurse Administration, 32*(3), 230–234.

Sewell, J. P., & Thede, L. Q. (2013). *Informatics and nursing* (4th ed.). Philadelphia, PA: Lippincott Williams & Wilkins.

American Organization of Nurse Executives (2013). AONE 2013 Year End Report. Retrieved from http://www.aone.org/docs/2013-year-end-report.pdf

UNIT III

CHAPTER 7

Systems Interoperability and Levels of Standardization

CHAPTER HIGHLIGHTS

This chapter discusses the following:

- How the use of information technologies, in designing support systems for healthcare practitioners, enables them to make collaborative decisions in the treatment of acutely or chronically ill patients in a timely and cost-effective manner
- How systems interoperability is making it easy and possible for healthcare practitioners to access individual patients' healthcare records online from many separate interoperable automated systems within an electronic record network
- How standards are helping prevent miscommunications and how, most importantly, interoperability is impossible without standardization
- How the diagnostic-related group (DRG) movement has included alternative healthcare, such as those provided by nurse practitioners, to the Alternative Billing Coding (ABC) set
- Student Experience: Necessity for Nursing Documentation to Contain Comparable Data

TYPES OF INFORMATICS

THE FIELD OF health informatics is broadly known as information science and the body of knowledge used to improve the accuracy, efficiency, and reliability of the entire healthcare delivery system, not only in the United States but in the majority of the Western world, including European and Asian countries. To have a health informatics discipline, information technology must be in place to allow the system to be used in improving the healthcare delivery system, wherever it is implored. A classic example of this can be seen in the use of information technology in designing support systems for healthcare practitioners, which will enable them to make collaborative decisions in the treatment of acute or chronically ill patients in a timely and cost-effective manner. Health informatics is a growing, dynamic, and wide field that permeates various disciplines, resulting in nursing informatics, consumer health informatics, radiology or imaging informatics, public health informatics, clinical health informatics, research informatics, pharmacy informatics, and bioinformatics. The applications of informatics also present in electronic health records, personal health records, and telemedicine.

SYSTEMS INTEROPERABILITY AND ITS CHALLENGES

The systems of electronic health records make it easy and possible for healthcare practitioners to access individual patients' healthcare records online from many separate, interoperable automated systems within an electronic record network. The interoperability of electronic health record systems makes patient's medical records portable and easily accessible to all healthcare providers since all patients are seen by many healthcare providers at any one given time (Brailer, 2005). A good example of the interoperability of the electronic health records is that it allows for the instantaneous sharing of health information among physicians, nurses, pharmacists, doctors' offices, and hospitals. More importantly, electronic health records provide an avenue for integration of individuals' health records with evidence-based clinical decision support, which often provides clinicians and healthcare providers with reminders and best clinical practice guidelines for treatment options. In addition, innovative research tools have been created to provide the primary care providers an avenue to review alternative diagnoses and improve access to critical and relevant evidence-based library resources without disrupting established workflows (Fowler, Yaeger, Yu, Doerhoff, Schoening, & Kelly (2014).

With the rapid and continual globalization of society today, it is necessary for us to realize the importance of the exchange of health information on a national level and throughout the world. The Office of the National Coordinator (ONC) has developed a framework project (the Standards and Interoperability Framework Consolidation Project) as an initiative to facilitate greater harmonization of standards to achieve greater health information exchange. It strives to achieve greater interoperability that will lead to an improved exchange of healthcare information while meeting the criteria for meaningful use (MU) (Alexander, 2011). This chapter enlightens its readers to a general pattern for developing standards, identify the need for standards, interpret the effects on standards of nursing at all levels of healthcare, identify organizations involved in setting standards at the international and the national level, and address the three types of interoperability: technical, semantic, and process.

In a nutshell, interoperability is the ability of two or more diverse systems or organizations to work together in the exchange of information. In healthcare, this correlates to the transmission and receipt of information to allow for the delivery of the highest level of healthcare to our communities and the world. Interoperability can most optimally be attained by complying with acceptable standards or by seamless third-party integration of multiple systems. This operates similar to the protocols of the Internet, which translates information. Of the three different types of interoperability, *technical* is the most functional. It is the basic transmission and reception of usable data. *Semantic* interoperability takes this to the next level in that it not only assures that the information is transmitted but communicated at the highest level.

> According to Raiford (2007) "semantic interoperability has huge implications for nurses who waste so much time asking patients questions they have answered 100 times before, but about which the data were not shared. Raiford further states when semantic interoperability is achieved between providers and between visits, nursing will be validating information, not collecting it

for another round of redundant data entry. The cornerstone of achieving semantic interoperability involve discussing IHE profiles, SNOMED, LOINC, HL7 V3, CDA, CCD, and ultimately certification by CCHIT." (Raiford & Sensmeier, 2007)

The aforementioned transactions can take place automatically and do not necessarily require human intervention. The third type is *process* interoperability and is the newest concept. This is what is mostly used in the work place, such as in electronic health records. Its goal is to provide user-friendly networks and effectiveness in actual use. Interoperability is vital to the success of computer networks and systems. Without this, it can become quite stressful, tedious, and time consuming to have to manually transcribe data to the different systems.

CODING SYSTEM

The healthcare common procedure coding system was implemented in the late 1970s and serves to standardize products and supplies such as prosthetics, ambulance services, durable medical equipment, and orthotics. To further the diagnostic related group (DRG) movement to include alternative healthcare, such as those provided by nurse practitioners, the Alternative Billing Coding (ABC) set was birthed. The ABC system is used for reimbursement of third parties as in alternative medicine and non-medical treatments and interventions. This provided the standard for billing for advanced practice nurses. Home healthcare agencies also have a standard of data elements that must be submitted for reimbursements. These study-driven set data elements allow for the measurement of patient outcomes and quality improvement. This process takes place through the Outcome and Assessment Information Set (OASIS). The OASIS provides feedback to home health providers in four areas: agency patient-related characteristics, potentially avoidable events, outcome-based quality improvements, and process quality measurements. It also allows for attention to other factors: functional status, health status, support systems, and environmental and socio-demographic data and also provide assistance in care planning for home health patients.

The endeavor of EHR for all Americans came to realization in 2014 and is still ongoing. There were several organizations, some of which have been mentioned previously, that were established to further this movement. The ONC supplies advisement on health information technology to the United States, Department of Health and Human Services and creates programs for them as well. The Health Information Technology for Economic and Clinical Health (HITECH) Act helps in dispersing funds from the ONC to advance information technology. The ONC, through HITECH, also provides state-level initiatives for healthcare, initiates the Nationwide Health Information Network (NHIN), assists in the Federal Health Architecture (FHA), implements health information technology adoption surveys, and provides clinical decision support (CDS). The state-level initiative to achieve interoperability is quite complex. The State Health Policy Consortium is focused on policy issues to allow for the exchange of health information across state lines, called the health information exchanges (HIEs). Alongside government bodies, the State Alliance is perusing best practices in the inter- and intrastate HIEs. There are other work groups involved in assuring privacy, security, policies, laws, and consistency in information exchange throughout the United States.

The work conducted by the National Health Information network, performed by government agencies, created the health information exchange organizations on the state, local, regional, and federal levels. These agencies are working to allow for the secure exchange of health information from one provider to another. The FHA is accountable for the integration of health information technologies for federal agencies that service the healthcare needs of the public. It supports federal government initiatives for disseminating health IT standards and has the authority to ensure a seamless exchange of health information technology between all levels of government and the private sector. The ONC conducts yearly surveys to assess and monitor the adoption of HIEs in private offices and in the hospital setting. The Clinical Decision Support organization delivers queues, called just in time, to assist healthcare providers, nurses, and patients in taking advantage of the use of health information systems in addition to the reduction of cost, increase in patient provider satisfaction, and improvement of efficiency. In 1949, the National Committee on Vital and Health Statistics was created by the Department of Health and Human Services in the collection of health data, statistics, and national health information policies (Sewell & Thede, 2013). Not included in the EHR movement is the U.S. Public Health Information Network (PHIN). This network strives to increase the use of standards, thus promoting the use and electronic exchange of health information.

The National Electronic Disease Surveillance System (NEDSS) also has a significant role in these efforts. It provides support and development of surveillance systems that are integrated to transmit health information securely and efficiently over the Internet. This activity allows for rapid identification of natural disease outbreaks or bioterrorism. There are several different simultaneous movements to standardize information technology and its terms. The Unified Medical Language System (UMLS) attempts to unify this process. It addresses three different but interrelated types of information. The first is the Metrathesaurus, which is simply a large vocabulary database. The second is the semantic network, which provides a unified systematic category to the large vocabulary database. The last is the SPECIALIST lexicon and lexical program. It comprises biomedical terms. The UMLS hope to link EHRs with biomedical literature in the future. Nursing care providers will be directly affected by the HIT standards and their initiatives. They will serve as a determination as to how the care provided is documented. They will also have a direct impact on healthcare policy. Nursing must maintain an active role in its contribution to the process of standardization and interoperability to ensure the best interest of the nursing and client relationship.

In conclusion, national and international standards are everywhere in our society. Although in its beginning stages, healthcare has now also developed and met standards and interoperability of its own. Currently, there are many systems that fail to interoperate. This increases the risk of potential lethal errors in patient care and hinders using integrated data in research. Government agencies on all levels have recognized this very problem and have put the man power and financial resources in place to overcome this extremely complex issue. While standards grounded in health information exchange may not be the only solution to national and worldwide healthcare reform, it certainly does assist in accomplishing the goal. According to Williams, Kontopantelis, Buchan, and Peek (2017),

> Given a completely error free terminology modelled as an ontology, and accurate clinical coding practices, there would perhaps be no need for the laborious process of constructing a code set. A researcher interested in type 2 diabetes would simply select all codes that were instances of that condition and they would be done. In practice this is not the case. Firstly, a terminology that does not support multiple inheritance will see codes for a condition occurring in separate branches of the tree requiring the researcher to exhaustively search across all terms without any form of filtering. Secondly, inaccurate coding practices necessitate that a researcher must also consider codes indicative of a covariate, for example using a code for "hypertension annual review" as a proxy for a patient with hypertension in the absence of a diagnostic code. Thirdly, terminologies may provide multiple ways to code the same concept. SNOMED is a good example of this where post-coordination allows, for example, at least four ways of describing acute appendicitis. This is beneficial to end users such as clinicians who can code information with their preferred method, however it is problematic for researchers when constructing code sets. Finally, any errors in the terminology whereby a code for a condition is in the wrong part of a tree again necessitate an exhaustive search. The larger the terminology, the greater the problem. The high proportion of papers from the UK using Read v2 codes identified by this review is perhaps indicative of that problem. ICD9, although used extensively around the world, is a relatively small terminology so the issue of creating code sets is not that great. Perhaps with the transition from ICD9 to ICD10 in the US we will start to see the issue of code set creation discussed more frequently in the literature. (p. 7)

LEVELS OF STANDARDIZATION IN NURSING

Standards are the minimum level of quality that are considered acceptable, and they help prevent miscommunication. Most importantly, interoperability is impossible without standardization. The idea of standards first began during the industrial revolution with the advent of the railroad system in the United States. The railroads set the first time zones, which were eventually accepted by state governments. Unfortunately, in healthcare, standards are being dictated by consumerism and great inefficiencies have resulted (Sewell & Thede, 2013). Standards affect everything that is done. With the recent implementation of electronic health records (EHR's) throughout the United States, it is imperative for nurses to be aware of the functioning of these systems and their role in the setting of the standards that will govern nursing practice. There are more than 60 groups charged with setting standards and eliminating inconsistencies. To have successful implementation of interoperable electronic health records, the work force must be properly trained in informatics.

The Health Information Technology for Economic and Clinical Health (HITECH), one of the groups involved in setting standards, has developed a program to rapidly prepare the workforce through education. There are six university base informatics roles that are supported: clinician or public health leader, health information management and exchange specialist, health information privacy and security specialist, research and development scientist, programmers and software engineers, and health information technology (HIT) subspecialist (Westra, 2011). Another group that plays an important role in establishing standards is the Health Information Technology Standards Panel (HITSP). "It is the national synchronization body responsible for the collaboration with the public and private sector to achieve a widely accepted and useful set of standards to enable wide spread interoperability among healthcare software applications" (Sensmeier & Alexander, 2009). They are in charge of several different tasks that include establishing HITSP interoperability specifications and promoting the acceptance, support, and deployment of HITSP interoperability specifications across the healthcare enterprise; facilitating the efforts of developing standards for organizations to maintain, revise, or develop new standards as required to support the HITSP interoperability specifications; and selecting and harmonizing standards. To summarize their tasks, "the primary goal of the organization is to harmonize and integrate diverse standards that will meet clinical and business needs for sharing information among organizations and systems, currently there are more than five hundred national and international organizations that are members of the HITSP" (Sensmeier & Alexander, 2009, (pp. 125–126)

International organizational involvement must be included in the collaboration and development of standards. The global nature of our society today demands the oversight of the International Organization of Standardization (ISO) and the International Electrotechnical Commission (IEC). These are the two groups involved in setting standards on an international level. The IEC is most concerned with setting the standards of equipment in hospital settings and the ISO sets the standards in all other areas. The ISO is a nonprofit organization that evolved more than 65 years ago and encompasses over 150 countries. Under the ISO, the reference terminology model was created. This model will assist in facilitating nursing documentation of diagnosis and intervention and allow for greater ease in mapping this information. Products used in the healthcare industry are also subject to standards. The IEC creates these standards, and its goal is to ensure that these products are efficient and satisfies the standards.

The American Society for testing and materials is an international entity that has major influence on the developers in the United States while acting as a reference to governments and corporations all over the world. Current-day concepts of epidemiology were established during the bubonic plague outbreaks of old England. At that time, the collection of data in regards to burials allowed for the ability to trend these outbreaks. Today, our world moves at a high rate of speed and is always seeking faster and more efficient means of carrying out everyday tasks. With this, the need to collect and disseminate healthcare information must also match this accelerated movement. It also further establishes the need for international healthcare standardization and international classification of disease standards. The World Health Organization (WHO) is responsible for the evaluation, update, and publication of the most current international statistical classification of disease and related health problems codes (ICD). These codes provide an in-depth listing of every known disease, track morbidity and mortality, and assign a specific code to each. These codes are utilized worldwide.

According to WHO (2018)

> "ICD-10 was endorsed in May 1990 by the Forty-third World Health Assembly. It is cited in more than 20,000 scientific articles and used by more than 100 countries around the world. A version of ICD-11 was released on 18 June 2018 to allow Member States to prepare for implementation, including translating ICD into their national languages. ICD-11 will be submitted to the 144th Executive Board Meeting in January 2019 and the Seventy-second World Health Assembly in May 2019 and, following endorsement, Member States will start reporting using ICD-11 on 1 January 2022" (p. 1)

In the United States these codes were initially used for billing purposes. Although they can also be used in nursing as a quality improvement tool to pool groups of patients with specific disease types together, they are not granular and do not retain enough data to be used in EHR. To make these codes more applicable, clinical modifications (CM) were created. This captures morbidity data from multiple sources. Also included under the umbrella of the WHO is the International Classification of Functioning, Disability and Health (ICF). The ICF codes, developed in 2001, are more qualitative in that they measure health and disability for both individuals and populations and the effect of disease on the holistic human experience. They serve to compliment the ICD-10 and provide further information on health disparities including functional status. The Health Level Seven (HL7) is an all-volunteer, nonprofit, international healthcare organization spearheaded by experts in healthcare informatics. Since its inception in the 1980s, it has channeled its energy toward the development of a framework of standards for functional and semantic interoperability of electronic healthcare information. The seven in its title indicates standards that are being set to the highest level. It simply means that it is focused on what data will be submitted and what data will be used. The various HL7 standards address a portion of this process and incorporate nurses' input in these efforts.

Another internationally and nationally recognized standards development group is the Digital Imaging and Communications in Medicine Organization (DICOM). Its focus is on setting and maintaining standards in the electronic transmission of digital images. This gives the opportunity for the exchange of digital medical images globally. Europe has its very own collaboration of standardizing bodies. The two entities are the European Committee for Standardization and the Comite European de Normalisation (CEN). The CEN has been given the authority, through European legislation, to make approved CEN standards the standards nationwide. This standard emphasizes the application of nursing terminology within healthcare information systems and within electronic messaging. The Systematized Nomenclature of Medicine-Clinical Terms (SNOMED) came about as a result of a collaborative effort between the National Health Service in the United Kingdom and the College of American Pathologists in the United States (Sewell & Thede, 2013).

The work of these organizations is done on a voluntary basis. Anyone who is a proven expert in the field can participate in these efforts. In the development of standards, there are four steps to be completed. These steps are similar to those in the nursing research process. In the first step there must be an identification of need. The second step requires the definition of the standard to be accomplished in technical terms and what action it will take to accomplish this goal. The third is the step that requires the greatest time investment and will be revisited on multiple occasions. This step is where literature review, collaborative discussions with other field experts, and research is conducted. This step will eventually produce defined terms or specification that is then tested in the last step. Returning to the third step may be necessary to refine these terms and specification and incorporate further input. The final step is where the group members vote on the standard. If agreed on, it will then be submitted to the organization for approval. If accepted by the organization, it then becomes standard. These steps are repeated when updates to a standard are required.

Due to the skyrocketing costs of healthcare, the need for the standardization of billing is an urgent issue. The attempts to standardize government payments to hospitals were initiated in the 1980s with the use of ICD codes and diagnosis-related groups (DRGs). The Center for Medicare and Medicaid Services created the DRGs as a means of tracking the use of hospital resources. However, it has since transformed into a system of prospective payments based on a category in which a patient is classified. Other countries have also followed suit in the development of DRG systems similar to that of the United States. Their codes are also used to determine healthcare pay outs. The original DRG model did not do well in including nursing services into its system. It was primarily focused on the medical aspect. Additional research has since created a system that takes nursing care into consideration.

According to Weaver, et 2005

> "The rise of evidence-base practice (EBP) as a standard for care delivery is rapidly emerging as a global phenomenon that is transcending political, economic and geographic boundaries. Evidence-based nursing (EBN) addresses the growing body of nursing knowledge supported by different levels of evidence for best practices in nursing care. Across all health care, including nursing, we face the challenge of how to most effectively close the gap between what is known and what is practiced. There is extensive literature on the barriers and difficulties of translating research findings into practical application. While the literature refers to this challenge as the "Bench to Bedside" lag, this paper presents three collaborative strategies that aim to minimize this gap. The *Bedside* strategy proposes to use the data generated from care delivery and captured in the massive data repositories of electronic health record (EHR) systems as empirical evidence that can be analyzed to discover and then inform best practice. In the *Classroom* strategy, we present a description for how evidence-based nursing knowledge is taught in a baccalaureate nursing program. And finally, the *Bench* strategy describes applied informatics in converting paper-based EBN protocols into the workflow of clinical information

systems. Protocols are translated into reference and executable knowledge with the goal of placing the latest scientific knowledge at the fingertips of frontline clinicians. In all three strategies, information technology (IT) is presented as the underlying tool that makes this rapid translation of nursing knowledge into practice and education feasible." (Weaver, et al 2005)

Student Experience: Necessity for Nursing Documentation to Contain Comparable Data

Mekonnem Dagmawit, RN, BSN

Nursing documentation is essential to everyday nursing practice. It includes all written and electronic data that reflect all aspects of patient care, from the history [and] recommended therapy to the treatment planning (ANA, 2010). Paper records allowed nurses and physicians to use terms they wanted and to write in their own manner and in purpose of data processing such collections of data needed to be translated by a third party into the same categories for comparison. Widespread use of electronic medical records demands all healthcare providers to use standardized language. It is often thought that standardization will impair the freedom of healthcare providers to accurately describe the patients' real status. In fact, most of the electronic systems that use standardized language offer the possibility to add narrative text. Moreover, a standardized approach in the era of electronic patient records can facilitate decision-making and increase the overall efficacy of healthcare system (Weaver, Delaney, Weber & Carr, 2010).

Standardized terminologies used by physicians have been developed during the 20th century, such as International Classification of Diseases and Related Health Problems (ICD), Diagnostic and Statistical Manual for Mental Health Disorders (DSM). The benefits of such standardized, internationally used and legally obliging classifications are obvious. They connect medical practice all over the world and enable the comparison of medical data across countries. Nursing data is usually not included in such systems. Without standardized terminology, nurses' contribution to the healthcare system cannot be recognized (Rutherford, 2008). Sharing data and communicating between nurses is limited due to the different data reporting styles and strategies and use of different terminology. Some studies indicate that 70% of all sentinel events are caused by lack of thorough and precise communication on patient handover (Alvarado, Lee, Christoffersen, Fram, Boblin, Poole, Lucas and Forsyth, 2006)

In order to be compared and processed, the data has to be standardized. Only standardized data can provide a realistic estimate of the healthcare quality. The inconsistency of data influences both national and international data processing and the final statistical results. Therefore, standardization of nursing language is of the utmost importance to the modern nursing practice. Several studies have proven that using standardized sets of data and standardized language improves patient safety and health outcomes, and therefore suggest[s] the development of the written and/or electronic forms that will be used in patient care (Chaudhry B1, Wang J, Wu S, Maglione M, Mojica W, Roth E, Morton SC, Shekelle PG. (2006).

Many think that one, internationally recognized, standardized nursing terminology should be used. That system should reflect the needs of all nursing subspecialties. Instead, the Committee for Nursing Practice Information Infrastructure of the American Nurses Association (ANA) has recognized twelve standardized terminology sets that support nursing practice (thirteen at first, one was retired) (ANA, 2012). These 12 standardized data sets are very heterogeneous: seven are nursing-specific, two cross-disciplinary and two are the so called minimum data sets. All these must be developed in a way that enables their use for electronic, computer-based records.

One of the barriers to introducing these standardized approaches to nursing care is the lack of education among nurses themselves. Thede and Schwiran (2011) have found that nearly one half of the nurses they have surveyed had no knowledge of any of the twelve ANA standardized terminology sets. This was true even for NANDA, which is the most recognizable among others, and it was not used in more than one third of the examined nurses. Therefore, educating nurses themselves is the first and the most important step in implementing these standards. The most widely used and best known are NANDA (Nursing Diagnoses, Definitions, and Classification), NIC (Nursing Interventions Classification) and NOC (Nursing Outcomes Classification). A higher level of organization is observed in SNOMED-CT (Systematized Nomenclature of Medicine-Clinical Terms) which enables interoperability between different nomenclatures.

One of the advantages of using standardized nursing languages is the better communication among nurses and other healthcare professionals not only inside the borders of the particular country, but also internationally. The use of such standardized systems can also help in better informing the nurses about the outdated or new procedures/concepts, and help them to make the decision regarding patient care based on evidence. A limited, but extensive list of possible choices, accessible by all the nurses around the world, enables the creation of the powerful database which can be further used to gather data regarding medical conditions themselves. For example, using standardized language as NIC can help us to quantitatively present the prevalence of certain measures taken under the specific circumstances. For example, Baena de Morales Lopes, M., Jose dos Reis, M., & Higa, R. (2004) have used this approach to identify the major nursing diagnoses and interventions in the case of rape.

Another benefit of using standardized nursing language is the increased visibility of nursing interventions. It is still common in many countries that nurses use informal writings or verbal communication instead of recording it as official patient record. Without being noted, the work of nurses is invisible. As Moss and Saba (2012) wrote, nursing care is one of the major determinants of healthcare cost and in order to be properly reimbursed, nursing work has to be visible, recognized and documented. As they are also accountable for what they do to the patients and the care they provide, it is necessary to record the activities that nurses take to treat the patient. For example, the use of NIC enables recording and recognizing intangible services that nurses often deliver such as emotional support. Emotional support is clearly identified in NIC, defined and described including all specific activities that lead to emotional support. In this manner, every service provided by the nurse can be recognized and documented.

The use of standardized nursing languages invariably improves patient care. One example is the use of Nursing Minimal Data Sets (NMDS). They represent the attempt to collect clinical data in a standardized and organized manner. The main purpose of NMDSs is to enable comparability among healthcare professionals of various clinical settings and geographical background. Benefits of using such standard sets are the access to comparable data, enhanced documentation on provided services, improved and easily retrievable data that can be used for quality surveillance, allowance for comparative research in nursing and contribution to the overall defining nursing as a research-based discipline. Standardized language in nursing also leads to greater adherence to standards of care (Rutherford, 2008). All interventions in NIC, for example, are evidence based, that is, based on relevant research that supports the current standards of patient management. Adhering to the standardized sets in nursing, one indirectly follows the recent and evidence-based standards in the health profession.

Evaluation of healthcare delivery is impossible without having comparable, standardized data. With the development of electronic databases this has become especially important because it facilitates the analysis of the data and enables the formation of large national and international databases which can be used for rapid analysis. Nursing competency can also be determined by using these standards. It can be done by simply observing the nurse in particular clinical settings and noting if the user follows the recommendations outlined in these standard sets. For example, NIC lists recommended activities for every intervention that is mentioned, and the knowledge and adherence to this standard can be easily determined only by observing the nurse's work at the bedside. It also supports nursing education. Nurse educators are advised to teach future nurses these standardized sets and to encourage young colleagues to use them in everyday practice, even in acute care settings. Implementing these standards in nursing education will improve the adherence to such sets in the future and invariably improve healthcare delivery. Research in nursing can also benefit from the usage of standardized language. The data is readily accessible and immediately available seconds after recording. This can lead to larger sample sizes in nursing research and more relevant research outcomes and conclusions (Rutherford, 2008).

It is impossible to introduce [a] standardized approach to nursing healthcare delivery overnight. One interesting example of the standardization and harmonization of nursing documentation is the Finnish model. It was based on Clinical Care Classification (CCC) and its use [was] introduced in Finland between 2005 and 2008.

It was designed in such a manner that reflects the five stages of nursing process: assessment, diagnosis, planning, implementation and evaluation (Weaver, 2010). The evaluation after a few years of use showed that this classification system was too complicated and difficult to understand and concluded that further efforts should be made in order to develop the model that is easy to use but also detailed and comparable (Nykanen, Kaipio, & Kuusisto (2012).

Great efforts are being made to integrate all above-mentioned standardized sets for nursing practice into one, universal standardized language. The future of nursing practice is tightly linked to the existence of a complete and comparable documentation and approach to nursing care.

References

Alvarado K., Lee R., Christoffersen E., Fram N., Boblin S., Poole N., Lucas J., & Forsyth S. (2006). Transfer of accountability: Transforming shift handover to enhance patient safety. *Healthcare Quarterly, 9,* 75–79.

American Nurses Association (ANA). (2010). Principles for nursing documentation: Guidance for registered nurses. Silver Spring, MD: Author.

American Nurses Association (ANA). (2012). *NCNQ, home of the NDNQI.* Retrieved from www.nursingworld.org/quality/

Baena de Morales Lopes, M., Jose dos Reis, M., & Higa, R. (2004). Nursing diagnosis: An aid when assisting the female victim of sexual violence. Paper presented at the NANDA, NIC, NOC 2004, Chicago, IL.

Brailer, D. (2005). Aims to Bring Down Barriers to EHRs: Says Oncologists Can Help. (2005). *Journal of oncology practice, 1*(2), 48–49.

Chaudhry B., Wang J., Wu S., Maglione M., Mojica W., Roth E., Morton S. C., & Shekelle, P. G. (2006). Systematic review: Impact of health information technology on quality, efficiency and costs of medical care. *Annals of Internal Medicine, 144,* 742–752. Retrieved from http://annals.org/article.aspx?articleid=723406

Fowler, S. A., Yaeger, L. H., Yu, F., Doerhoff, D., Schoening, P., & Kelly, B. (2014). Electronic health record: integrating evidence-based information at the point of clinical decision making. *Journal of the Medical Library Association: JMLA, 102*(1), 52–5.

Moss, J. & Saba, V. (2012). Costing nursing care: Using the clinical care classification system to value nursing intervention in an acute-care setting. *CIN: Computers, Informatics, Nursing, 36*(11). Retrieved from http://journals.lww.com/cinjournal/pages/default.aspx

Nykanen, P., Kaipio, J., & Kuusisto, A. (2012). Evaluation of the national nursing model and four nursing documentation systems in Finland—lessons learned and directions for the future. *International Journal of Medical Informatics, 81*(8): 507–520. doi:10.1016/j.ijmedinf.2012.02.003

Raiford, R., & Sensmeier, J. (2007). Semantic interoperability in HIT-finally! Get ready! It is coming soon to electronic health records. *CIN: Computers, Informatics, Nursing, 25*(5), 310.

Rutherford, M. (2008). Standardized nursing language: What does it mean for nursing practice? *Online Journal of Issues in Nursing, 13*(1).

Sensmeier, J., & Alexander, G. (2009). Leveraging standards to achieve interoperability: An update on the healthcare information technology standards panel. *CIN: Computers, Informatics, Nursing, 27*(2), 125–126.

Sewell, J. P., & Thede, L. Q. (2013). *Informatics and nursing* (4th ed.). Philadelphia, PA: Lippincott Williams & Wilkins.

Thede, L., & Schwiran, P. (2011). Informatics: The standardized nursing terminologies: A national survey of nurses' experiences and attitudes. *Online Journal of Issues in Nursing, 16*(2). doi:10.3912/OJIN.Vol16No02InfoCol01

Weaver C., Delaney C., Weber P., Carr R. (2010). *Nursing and informatics for the 21st century* (2nd ed.). New York: NY, CRC Press.

Weaver, C. A., Warren J. J., Delaney, C. (2005). Bedside, classroom and bench: Collaborative strategies to generate evidence-based knowledge for nursing practice. *International Medical Informatics Association, Nursing Informatics* Volume 74, Issues 11-12, December 2005, Pages 989–999 https://doi.org/10.1016/j.ijmedinf.2005.07.003

Westra, B. (2011). HITECH university-based training. *CIN: Computers, Informatics, Nursing, 29*(4), 263–264.

Williams, R., Kontopantelis, E., Buchan I., & Peek, N. (2017). Clinical code set engineering for reusing EHR data for research: A review. *Journal of Biomedical Informatics, 70*(2017) 1–13.

World Health Organization (2018). ICD-11 is here, history of ICD. Retrieved from https://www.who.int/classifications/icd/en/International Journal of Medical Informatics Volume 74, Issues 11-12, December 2005, Pages 989–999

CHAPTER 8

Data Mining and Knowledge Discovery

CHAPTER HIGHLIGHTS

This chapter discusses the following:

- How data are generated including assigning field names, recognizing data types, creating tables, determining primary key components, entering relevant data in tables, creating as well as designing forms, understanding queries, and generating reports for the final assessment
- How data modeling and logical design are used in recognizing the entity of classes that are represented in a particular database along with forming effective interrelations between the pairs of these entities
- How examples of data analysis and queries are generated from the national inpatient stay dataset on the outcome of inpatients hospitalized with both diabetes and myocardial infarction
- How cleaned data could be transformed into information after interpretation, which could lead to knowledge that could be visualized and presented—not forgetting that accumulation of knowledge over time results into experience and wisdom
- How the diagnostic related group (DRG) movement has included alternative healthcare, such as those provided by nurse practitioners, to the alternative billing coding (ABC) set

DATABASE CREATION

THERE ARE TWO separate steps in creating a database. One of the steps in forming a database includes the following: creation of the database, defining the views as well as the fields in the database, setting strong permissions in the database, and creating database reports, which is optional. Other steps used in creating a database encompass analyzing data, categorizing data, segregating tables, assigning field names, recognizing data types, creating tables, determining primary key components, entering relevant data in tables, creating as well as designing forms, understanding queries, and generating along with designing reports for the final assessment. In summary, there are a few basic rules for data creation as itemized by Russell Dyer in Chapter 4 of *Creating Databases and Tables*, as depicted below:

- The number of tables to include in your database, as well as the table names
- For each table, the number of columns it should contain, as well as the column names
- For each column, what kind of data is to be stored

(Dyer, 2018, https://www.oreilly.com/library/view/learning-mysql-and/9781449362898/ch04.html)

TABLE 8.1

INSURANCE	COMORBIDITIES	ADMISSION TYPE	TREATMENT PROCEDURES	WEIGHT
Medicare	NULL	Emergency	NULL	NULL
Medicaid	NULL	Emergency	NULL	NULL
Medicaid	NULL	Emergency	NULL	134.249
Medicare	401.9	Emergency	NULL	159
Medicaid	440.9	Emergency	NULL	119
Medicaid	401.9	Emergency	NULL	130.312
Medicaid	443.9	Emergency	NULL	130.312
NULL	NULL	Emergency	NULL	400.003
Medicaid	NULL	Emergency	0.66	189
Medicaid	401.9	Emergency	NULL	160.001
Medicaid	401.9	Emergency	NULL	160.001
Medicaid	401.9	Emergency	NULL	160.001
Medicaid	401.9	Emergency	NULL	160.001
Medicaid	NULL	Emergency	NULL	156
Self-pay	401.9	Emergency	NULL	166.061
Self-pay	401.9	Emergency	NULL	166.061
Medicaid	NULL	NULL	0.66	184.313
Medicaid	NULL	NULL	0.66	184.313
Medicaid	401.9	NULL	NULL	239.001
Medicaid	NULL	Emergency	NULL	203
Medicaid	401.9	Emergency	NULL	227.001
Medicaid	401.9	Emergency	NULL	155.124

Medicaid	401.9	Emergency	NULL	426.001
Medicaid	401.9	Emergency	NULL	94.2489
Others	401.9	NULL	NULL	160.001
Medicaid	401.9	Emergency	NULL	200.563
NULL	401.9	Emergency	NULL	131.187
Medicaid	NULL	Emergency	NULL	151
Medicaid	401.9	Emergency	NULL	294.001

Sample of Mini Database: Courtesy of Dr. Okunji's unpublished urban hospital data generated from EHR/EMR systems (2016)

Apart from the discussed steps, there also exist certain significant aspects that are required to be taken into account while creating a database. In this similar concern, these aspects comprise adoption along with execution of a database wizard, downloading a particular template, and implementing a database object. The aspect of a database wizard aids in creating a database through generating a predetermined set of tables, forms, queries as well as reports. It is worth mentioning that the facet concerning downloading a template is duly considered to be one of the quickest ways of creating a particular database. In addition, the adoption as well as the execution of a database object helps to create a database by customizing a table and designing a query, among others (Microsoft Corporation, 2013). Thus, on the basis of the discussion, it can be affirmed that the aforementioned aspects play an imperative role in creating a database by a considerable level.

RELEVANT EXPERIENCE AND EXPERTISE OF THE AUTHOR

In this section, data are presented that demonstrate that the author of this book has experience with clinical and population-based research. In 2008, the author planned, implemented, and completed a nation-wide study on the outcomes of patients with DMl in nonfederal hospitals for discharges in the year 2006. Her dissertation study drew on data from the 2006 Nationwide Inpatient Sample, Healthcare Cost and Utilization Project (HCUP), and Agency for Healthcare Research and Quality (Okunji, Afghani, Hegamin, & Gomez, 2012). Three articles were published from this effort (Okunji, Afghani, Hegamin, & Gomez, 2012; Okunji & Gomez, 2014; Okunji, Afghani, & Gomez, 2012) and two intramural grants with one fellowship funded in part by NIH and Research Office, Howard University.

KNOWLEDGE DISCOVERY

This section will also discuss methods of discovering knowledge in both relational and large databases. Prior to identifying the methods of discovering knowledge in both relational and large databases, it is quite essential to comprehend the inner meaning of knowledge discovery in databases (KDD). KDD is fundamentally described as an exploratory as well as an automatic study, along with modeling of huge data repositories.

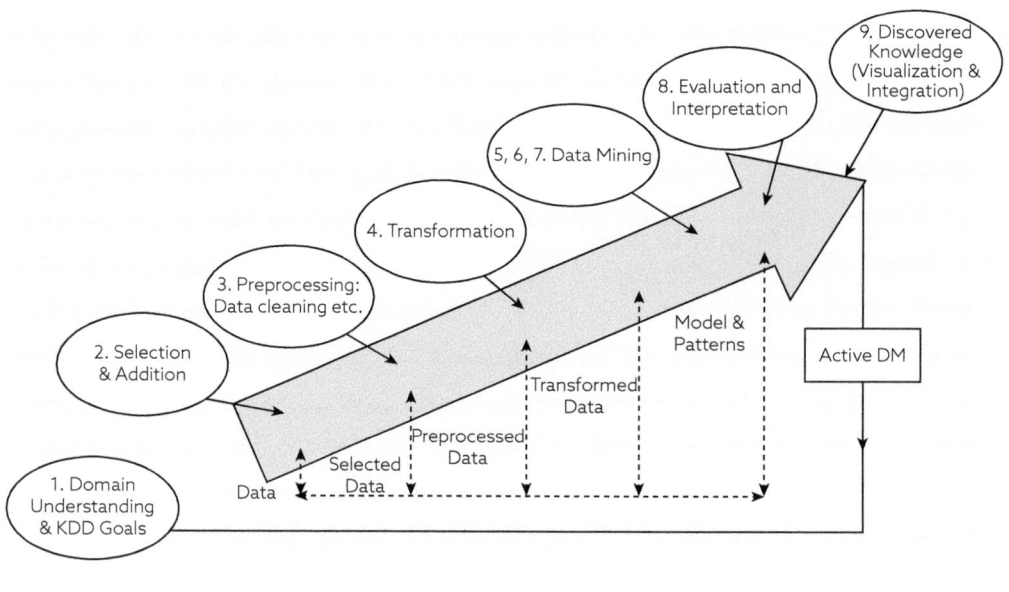

FIGURE 8.1

Source: (Maimon & Rokach, 2009).

It is often duly considered as a sort of organized procedure that recognizes novel, useful, understandable, and valid patterns from large and composite data sets.

According to Maimon & Rokach, 2009,

> "Since the information age, the accumulation of data has become easier and storing it inexpensive. It has been estimated that the amount of stored information doubles every twenty months. Unfortunately, as the amount of electronically stored information increases, the ability to understand and make use of it does not keep pace with its growth. Data Mining is a term coined to describe the process of sifting through large databases for interesting patterns and relationships. The studies today aim at evidence-based modeling and analysis, as is the leading practice in medicine, finance and many other fields. The data availability is increasing exponentially, while the human processing level is almost constant. Thus, the gap increases exponentially. This gap is the opportunity for the KDD\DM field, which therefore becomes increasingly important and necessary." (p. 2)

The following graphical representation depicts the methods of discovering knowledge in both relational and large databases.

On the basis of this pictorial illustration, it can be affirmed that there are several methods of discovering knowledge in both relational and large databases. In this regard, the methods have been described in the following discussion in an ascending order. Domain understanding and KDD goals build a setting for comprehending what should be done by adopting as well as executing effective decisions. Moreover, the method defines the objectives of end users and vitally enables them to learn about the setting wherein the procedure of knowledge discovery would occur. Selection and addition come after the determination of the KKD goals; this method identifies what sorts of data are accessible, along with acquiring extra necessary data and integrating all data into one specific data set for effective knowledge discovery. This method is quite important to discover knowledge in both relational and large databases because the procedure concerning knowledge development largely relies on selected necessary data by a certain degree (Maimon & Rokach, 2006).

DATA LABELS AND COMPUTER LANGUAGES

Meanwhile, prior to identifying and differentiating the methods of viewing data in a particular database, it is quite indispensable to acquire a brief idea about different levels of data that need to be viewed. In this regard, the various data labels comprise schema, both physical and subschema. Schema represents an overall logical outlook or view of the interrelations amid data in a specific database. On the other hand, subschema denotes a logical outlook of data affiliation required to develop the application programs of the specific end users. Finally, physical data level signifies identification about how data is physically stored, arranged, and accessed in various devices of a particular computer system. After acquiring a brief understanding about various data levels, numerous methods can apparently be viewed to be largely accessible for viewing diverse sorts of data in a particular database. In this similar concern, the various methods of viewing data in a database comprise structured query languages (SQL), data modeling or logical design, normalization, and physical design. It is strongly believed that with the aforementioned methods, users can view data in a database by a significant level. A detailed analysis and differentiation of these methods will be discussed next.

SQL is regarded as an international standard-based access language, which is typically used for defining as well as manipulating data in databases. The notion of data modeling or logical design denotes recognizing the entity of classes that are represented in a particular database along with forming effective interrelations between pairs of these entities. The term "normalization" is often regarded as the generalization of the logical outlook of data in relation to large databases. The aspect of logical design represents answering the queries that rise by typical databases. To differentiate the methods of viewing data in a database, it can be stated that there exists a vital demarcation between SQL and data modeling or logical design. In this regard, the demarcation lies in reference to the fact that SQL is broadly used in maintaining large databases, whereas data modeling or logical design is applied in relational databases. Perhaps, it is important to note here that one of the main differences between normalization and physical design is that the former simplifies the logical representation of data in both relational and large databases and the latter tends to answer the queries of the databases.

In conclusion, as this section has shown, the collecting, storing, and sharing of patient's information through database has proven to be an effective aid for providing adequate care to patients. Through databases, physicians, nurses, institutions, and health systems are able to share patients' diagnoses in a timely manner. The ability to have such information as quick as possible has resulted in the saving of many lives and in better management of time, energy, and resources. It has reduced the risk in medication complications since all authorized users would be seeing the medication that has been given, when, and those who needed to be given it at a given time. Although a database is not a perfect technology, and while it has its disadvantages, there is a strong belief and encouragement that its continued use in the healthcare system has benefits that outweigh its shortcomings. The author's experience in working with data analytics was shared as well.

References

Dyer, R. J. T (2018). Learning MySQL and MariaDB, Chapter 4. Creating Databases and Tables. Retrieved from https://www.oreilly.com/library/view/learning-mysql-and/9781449362898/ch04.html

Maimon, O., & Rokach, L. (2009). The KDD process. *Introduction to Knowledge Discovery in Databases in book Data mining and knowledge discovery handbook*, 1–17. Retrieved from https://www.researchgate.net/publication/225835494_Chapter_1_-_Introduction_to_Knowledge_Discovery_in_Databases

Microsoft Corporation. (2013). *Create an access database*. Retrieved from http://office.microsoft.com/en-us/access-help/create-an-access-database-HP005187442.aspx

Okunji P. O., Afghani A., Hegamin, A., & Gomez F. (2012). Comparative statistical analysis of in-patients with diabetic myocardial infarction: Patient length of stay. *Internet Journal of Allied Health Sciences and Practice, 10*(2), 1–7.

Okunji P. O., Afghani A., & Gomez F. (2012). Exploring the disparities in healthcare outcomes of inpatient diabetic myocardial infarction transfers in non-federal hospitals. *Journal of the National Black Nurses Association, 23*(1), 29–33.

Okunji, P. O., & Gomez, F. (2014). Effects of patients and hospital characteristics on myocardial infarction mortality: Health disparity outcomes. *Association of Black Nursing Faculty Journal, 25*(1), 13–18.

Oracle. (2011). HITECH's challenge to the health care industry [white paper]. Retrieved from https://www.oracle.com/technetwork/database/security/owp-security-hipaa-hitech-522515.pdf

Sewell, J. P., & Thede, L. Q. (2013). *Informatics and nursing* (4th ed.). Philadelphia, PA: Lippincott Williams & Wilkins

Figure Credits

Fig. 8.1: Adapted from Lior Rokach and Oded Maimon, Data Mining with Decision Trees, Theory and Applications. Copyright © 2007 by World Scientific.

CHAPTER 9

Data and Evidence-Based Research in Nursing

CHAPTER HIGHLIGHTS

This chapter discusses the following:

- Why the American Association of College of Nursing recommends that nursing curriculum include information-seeking, sorting and selecting, critical thinking, and healthcare technologies
- How clients could misdiagnose themselves from information accessed about their condition and do not discuss it with their healthcare provider, but use it in making decisions about their treatment
- Why the Joint Commission statement also highlights the fundamental right of the patient relating to evidence–based practice to receive information in such a way that they can understand it
- How the HITECH is driving the implementation of next-generation health IT and big data systems through the mandated meaningful use (MU) criteria for electronic health records (EHRs)
- How it is imperative that providers and students should be able to evaluate Internet health information and differentiate what is scholarly publication from what is not to be information and health literate for consumers
- Challenges facing the nursing profession from being evidenced-based savvy
- Students research experience through evidenced-based systemic reviews

ONE OF THE currently-used phrases in nursing is evidence-based practice (EBP), which is a critical mandate to ensure that most nursing interventions are based on the most current, and reliable evidence (Earle-Foley, 2011). The Canadian Nurses Association has called for the use of an evidence base in decision making in order to increase positive outcomes for patients, improve clinical practice, achieve cost effective nursing care and ensure accountability and transparency in decision making (CNA, 2002). Due to the rapid changes in healthcare development and information technology, information and health literacy skills are necessary for nurses and other healthcare professionals. By the same token, the American Association of Colleges of Nursing (AACN) recommends that nursing curriculum include information seeking, sorting and selecting, critical thinking, and healthcare technologies.

There is a difference between the knowledge found in online library databases and knowledge found using the Internet. Websites contain information that may be highly significant but may be trivial and obscene and without quality control or any guide to quality. It is difficult to utilize information retrieved from the Internet on face value due to poor quality. Librarians select materials necessary for academics by applying and using a set of explicit and meaningful selection criteria. Library guides and tutorial guides are needed for technology development. The improvement of nurses relies on demonstration of digital library competency.

The era of the Internet has brought about innumerable positive changes in people's way of life. In the 21st century, more and more people are seeking ways to improve their health outcome. Prior to this era of enhanced computer usage, people had depended on their personal care provider for information about their health. In those days, a patient was not even allowed to see his or her medical record. Health information was held uptight in research centers, school libraries, and journals. Now, Internet had exposed health information that was kept from the general public. With the introduction of the World Wide Web, non-health workers can obtain any information related to their health condition. Even research institutions are granting access to healthcare information and knowledge. One could go to public library to use computer in case one did not have access to the Internet. Consumers are being proactive and seeking information and services to improve their health outcome. However, the public needs assistance to effectively evaluate and use the most updated health information. According to Lydia M., internet should be evaluated with the following six (6) criteria: authority, accuracy, objectivity, currency, coverage, and appearance. Each criterium has several questions to be asked as depicted in the below table. The more questions to which you can answer "yes," the more likely the website is one of quality.

RISK OF SELF DIAGNOSIS

Today, consumers take the responsibility of their own care and can access healthcare-related information. Given the amount of information and new knowledge, it is impossible for healthcare providers to keep up with all the new technology. With the advancement in technology, most consumers are savvy. They search the Web for information and conditions they have. They often arrive at their office visits with printouts of information, which may result in conflicts because the provider may not be aware of the information. This certainly opens an avenue for discussion. One serious problem to note is that clients may access information about their condition and do not discuss it with their healthcare provider but use it in making decisions about their treatment. It is always good to ask a client if he or she has accessed any information and hopefully this will start a conversation, which will lead to better understanding.

E-LIBRARY AND HEALTH LITERACY

Healthcare professionals need to be fortified—be one step ahead of the game to guide consumers in making the right decisions about the care they receive. Healthcare workers must have information literacy, health literacy, and information technology skills to find and explain reliable health information for improved patient outcome. Information literacy is the ability to identify the need for information, to search and locate the information, to synthesize the information, and to use the information to solve problems. And relating to information literacy is health literacy, which is the extent of the quest and ability of

TABLE 9.1 Internet Evaluation Criteria

AUTHORITY	ACCURACY	OBJECTIVITY	CURRENCY	COVERAGE	APPEARANCE
Is it clear who is responsible for the contents of the page? Is there a way of verifying the legitimacy of the organization, group, company or individual? Is there any indication of the author's qualifications for writing on a particular topic? Is the information from sources known to be reliable?	Are the sources for factual information clearly listed so they can be verified in another source? Is the information free of grammatical, spelling, and other typographical errors?	Does the content appear to contain any evidence of bias? Is there a link to a page describing the goals or purpose of the sponsoring organization or company? If there is any advertising on the page, is it clearly differentiated from the informational content?	Are there dates on the page to indicate when the page was written, when the page was first placed on the Web, or when the page was last revised?	Are these topics successfully addressed, with clearly presented arguments and adequate support to substantiate them? Does the work up-date other sources, substantiate other materials you have read, or add new information? Is the target audience identified and appropriate for your needs?	Does the site look well organized? Do the links work? Does the site appear to be well maintained?

Source: Olson L. M (2018). Evaluating Internet Sources, A Library Resource Guide: https://library.nmu.edu/guides/userguides/webeval.htm

an individual to obtain, assimilate, and use common health information and services to make positive health decisions. There is no doubt that health literacy is important and beneficial to everyone. The problem is the quality and availability of the information and the ability of the client to understand it. Health literacy has been defined as the degree to which individuals have the capacity to obtain, process and understand basic health information and services needed to make appropriate health decisions US Department of Health and Human Services (2000). Health literacy involves the ability to understand and read instructions, medication brochures, doctor's directions, and consent forms and the ability to navigate the complex health system.

Both information and health literacy are learned processes that need to be continually maintained. They require continuous practicing over time in different settings to master the act. Information technology skills, on the other hand, are the ability to utilize computer skills in daily operations, knowing the component of computer software, hardware applications, and the ability to use updated information technology to solve problems. The three kinds of nursing knowledge important for information technology skills include present skills, information technology fundamental concepts, and cognitive ability.

HEALTH NUMERACY

Similar to health literacy is also health numeracy. Health numeracy is the ability of the consumer to understand and interpret numerical information to make effective health decisions. It does not correlate with the educational level or the ability to read; for example, a diabetic patient required to take insulin needs to understand the treatment, comply with the regimen, and make insulin dosage decisions based on a glucometer. This process requires the ability of the client to understand numbers, calculations, and follow directions and read labels. Timing of medication can also pose a problem without health literacy and numeracy skills, especially when they are several medications with different time schedules. Poor outcomes have been noted with anticoagulation control and history of asthma hospitalizations. This lack of knowledge can create difficulties when clients have to calculate dosages. Research has found that many consumers lack basic probability skills, which makes it difficult to manage health problems.

Online support groups have so many advantages over face-to-face groups. Members can participate any time or day without restriction to time, geography, or space. The messages can be carefully thought out and edited before posting. One of the advantages is that there is no monopoly. Participants can come from diverse groups and with different perspectives, opinions, and information sources. Most of the groups are anonymous, which is helpful in discussing sensitive or embarrassing situations. One disadvantage is that an individual may be spending a lot of time online alone when the company of others is needed.

Hospitals and other healthcare institutions provide online support services for their patients with varied content, which may include information about the organization, a map and directions to the agency, a list of services offered by the organization, and other organizational information for marketing purposes. The healthcare institutions post information related to their specialty. They may even develop a site with a specific condition, which will function as an extranet, and access may be restricted to clients only. The site may not be tied to an electronic health record (EHR). Healthcare organizations should have written guidelines for the use of information provided on their website, privacy and security issues and rights and responsibility of users and providers should also be addressed. Patient input may become part of their health record and they must be notified of such practice.

In conclusion, the introduction of e-health has opened a new means of providing quality care. According to Gulzar, Khoja, and Sajwani (2013),

> The satisfaction of consumers is increased due to increased access and quality care available in their environment. More importantly, nurses see ehealth as a solution to reduce professional isolation since they are now exposed to new knowledge through tele-consultation and e-learning. It is important to introduce e-health as part of nursing practice and nursing curriculum. Overall e-health is useful and challenging in terms of providing patient care. Ongoing training is required to help nurses' confidence and support their professional development." (Gulzar et al., 2013)

Consumer informatics has developed along with the empowerment of the consumers. Consumers now have access to information that ordinarily was not available to them. This availability of information hopefully will improve the relationship between healthcare provider and consumer. This continued growth would require greater attention to how health literacy and health numeracy affect client teaching. Nurses will have to add websites and various search engines as part of client teaching.

Healthcare agencies will use patient portals to provide consumer education, some of which may be restricted or individualized for their clients. These portals, on one hand, will serve as a marketing strategy to attract consumers. The role of nurses as well as nursing interventions will change over time to accommodate client teaching, which will include installing a computer, referring clients to places where basic computer skills are taught, and providing help with clients who are physically challenged. With this improvement in technology, e-health and telehealth opportunities are endless, especially to nurses. It has been proven to contain valuable information for patient care and disaster care. E-health and telehealth are still evolving and continue to have major concerns that hopefully will be addressed in the future. It is important to note some of the security issues and be prepared to deal with the problems as they occur.

Medicare has started reimbursing telehealthcare in the United States; however, Medicaid, which is controlled at the state level, has variations in reimbursement. There are still technical difficulties with the new technology, which can only improve with time. Telehealth will definitely change the way healthcare is provided; it will also provide more opportunities for nurses. The overall care will be guided to preventive care, which helps reduce emergency room visits and hospital readmissions.

INFORMATION RELIABILITY

According to Sewell and Thede (2013), out of approximately 80% of people who use the Internet, about 68% of them who had chronic disease looked for health information relating to the diseases. And out of 85 million American people who had looked for health information, only 15% checked for the information's origin, and when it was written.

There was no way to validate the reliability of the information as well (Sewell & Thede, 2013). The morbidity and mortality rates from diabetes and cardiovascular disorders among disadvantaged minorities and the underserved continue to increase. Advances in information technology (IT) have great potential to aid understanding of, and ultimately ameliorate the role of, healthcare inequality in minorities and the underserved (Calman, Kitson, & Hauser, 2007; Gibbons, 2005; Ketcham, Lutfey, Gerstenberger, Link, & McKinlay, 2009). The care delivery inefficiencies from individual providers have resulted in a large fraction of the $600–850 billion surplus in healthcare spending (Foster, 2016). The Health Information Technology for Economic and Clinical Health (HITECH) and the Affordable Care Act (ACA) are enabling private healthcare systems that provide for standards of healthcare record interoperability and will enable the use of big data tools to provide innovations in the use of technologies to reduce cost and improve the quality of healthcare. While both these acts are important to the current national effort at healthcare reform, it is primarily the HITECH, which was not part of the Supreme Court case, that is driving the implementation of next-generation health IT and big data systems through the mandated meaningful use (MU) criteria for electronic health records (EHRs). EHRs describing patient treatments and outcomes are presently an underutilized source of health information. Biomedical informatics is the discipline that seeks to apply computer and communication technology to improve health. Special efforts are made by informatics research training programs to recruit individuals from underrepresented racial and ethnic groups, individuals with disabilities, and those from economically, socially, culturally, or educationally disadvantaged backgrounds, into careers in biomedical informatics (United States National Library of Medicine, 2016).

INFORMATION LITERACY DEVELOPMENT

Healthcare information and technology is a dynamic movement; therefore, healthcare professionals must be abreast of events to update their skills to be proficient. To facilitate this process, the American Association of College of Nursing recommends that nursing education programs include effective ways for looking, grouping, choosing, thinking out of the box, and understanding information and information technology.

By the same token, the majority of other nursing organizations such as Technology Informatics Guiding Education Reform (TIGER) and National League for Nursing (NLN) have recognized and encouraged teaching informatics in nursing programs. Also, the Joint Commission statement also highlights the fundamental right of the patient, relating to evidence-based practice, to receive information in such a way that they can understand it. Also, the American Library of Information inferred that any literate person also know the six competencies, ranging from being able to know the amount of information required to comprehend the ethical, legal, financial, interpersonal ramifications of the information in question (Sewell & Thede, 2013)

Due to the numerous recognitions and encouragements and particularly from American Nurses Association recommendations, the nursing programs are beginning to incorporate fundamental information searches for evidence-based practice into knowledge domain and clinical practice. According to research, exposing student nurses to informatics earlier in their programs yield better results. In fact, there is a big difference between the masters and PhD candidates who were exposed to early Web-based information skills as evidence-based practice (EBP) and those who did not have early exposure. Those who were introduced to information literacy domain earlier on had ample time to build, test, and retain their knowledge.

This suggests that nurses must have clinical experience, develop fundamental research skills, and synthesize, differentiate and apply the knowledge to practice. So, it is imperative that nurses be exposed to information knowledge domain and evidence-based practice in various research settings earlier in their career to retain information and be able to help patients make informed health decisions. The knowledge also will aid the nurse in discussing and communicating evidence-based practice in the work place.

In addition, the knowledge acquired will equip the nurse in critical thinking, intellectual commitment to understanding situations, and applying information to generate knowledge for better result and outcome. The knowledge generated will assist the nurse better in informing patients from their point of admission to the discharge process, depending on the severity of the illnesses. The knowledge will enhance effective communication about the preventive and health promotion attitudes and less frequent hospital admissions. These in turn will decrease the financial burden for patients as well as the government and boost the overall health of the nation.

STEPS TO EVALUATING NURSING INFORMATION

The national statistic on health literacy indicated that about 90 million Americans with below average health literacy skills to comprehend and comply with their health instructions. Over 66% of adults have minimal literacy skills, minorities, particularly Hispanics (50%), Black (40%), and Asians (33%) (NCES, 2015). Another study by the Health Information Literacy Research Project also revealed that the more illiterate the consumer is, the more he or she will utilize the health system service and be less likely to utilize health preventive services. The research noted that improved health literacy will help patients positively comply with their specific disease modality (Shipman, Kurtz-Rossi, & Funk, 2009). The health illiteracy is such a national concern that health communication and health information technology, its goals, overviews, and benefits, are among the topics and objectives of Healthy People 2020 (ODPHP, 2010)

Furthermore, Internet health information on the Web is proliferating. For a nurse to obtain health information on the Internet website, he or she must follow stipulated professional standards for Web check lists which include the following:

- Origin of the article, who wrote the article, the credentials, any contact information, and if the author can be easily reached
- Who sponsored the article, who they affiliate with, if they have any commercial funding that may result in conflict of interest
- The authenticity of the information, the intent, and potential bias in the information
- Privacy of the statement meeting the established standards

Again, nursing Internet knowledge should focus on issues that enhance our professionalism such as laws, rules, and regulations, relating to our organizations such as the National Council of State Board of Nursing (NCSBN), the National Council Licensure Examination (NCLEX), the Joint Commission and Center for Medicare and Medicaid Services rules and regulations, the government health and disease entities such as the Center for Disease Control and Prevention (CDC), the National Institute for Health (NIH), continuing education resources issues, and evidence-based nursing resources.

WHAT SCHOLARLY PUBLICATIONS ARE AND WHAT THEY ARE NOT

Nursing research as well as other disciplines should utilize authentic reliable articles in their research. Scholarly journals, also known as academic, professional, or peer-reviewed articles, are written by scholars who have in-depth knowledge of the subject matter in the field. The authors must have established credentials. Articles or journals undergo a rigorous peer review process whereby if article is accepted by the editor in the first place, it is then given to other scholars in the same field to review for validity. Before the article is given to the peers, the author's name will be removed to avoid any bias. After the manuscript is reviewed and accepted, it is then given back to the author to do a final review and edit before the article can be published. Such articles are usually directed to fellow professionals or students in the same field. The scholarly article often reports previous research or experiments, or the author may shed new light on the subject. The scholarly articles have footnotes and bibliographies. The publishers are usually the professional publishers. Such journals include but are not limited to *American Journal for Nurses (AJN), Online Journal of Nursing Informatics (OJNI), Free Medical Journals, Biomed Central,* and *Cumulative Index to Nursing and Allied Health Literature (CINAHL)*. Access to such articles are open but may require that users log in. It is essential that nurses know that scholarly journals are written by qualified nurses who have expertise in the subject area. This is the major difference that sets scholarly nursing journals or any other professional journal apart (Sewell & Thede, 2013)

On the other hand, the magazines, newspapers, newsletters, and/or website articles, such as EzineArticles, could be written by reporters, journalists, or freelance writers. They are usually written with no nursing expertise for the general public. Such information may or may not be cited. Whereas scholarly information may appear serious with graphs and the like, the freelance aspect of newsletters or newspapers may appear colorful with pictures. Such information sometimes may lack quality. They are sometimes not updated regularly and are not cited or archived. Some online journals allow for full-text access but require fees.

Evidenced-based practice is a process that utilizes the best research outcome and the best clinical outcome, along with patient's response to reach the best clinical cost-effective decision. Evidence-based practice is the gold standard for future nursing actions. It is a process that revolves around the patient. The evidence-based library resources give comprehensive amount of in-depth resources that assist users in learning, educating, and implementing evidence-based practice. An example is the Cochrane Library. The library also provides online resources including grants, research journals, and list of database resources unlike the online evidence-based resources that provide a starting point for nursing and healthcare professionals who are beginning to learn evidence-based practice. For example, Sigma Theta Tau International is the best evidence-based online database resource.

To identify online evidence-based resources, one had to first identify from which part of the evidence-based practice topic he or she wants information or resources. For example, if looking for information on history, definition, or challenges, then one had to type "evidenced-base practice + the topic - definition, history or challenges." The website address or the universal resource locator (URL) will appear. The Internet has a vast array of powerful information to integrate evidence-based practice. These include the United States government through National Guideline Clearinghouse (NGC) and the website www.ahrq.gov/news/infoqual.htm.

FACTORS IMPENDING ADOPTION OF EVIDENCE-BASED PRACTICE IN NURSING

- Lack of resources: It takes quite a lot of money to implement evidence-based practice (EBP), and if the facility does not have the funds, it would not think of EBP. There are grants for the implementation for EBP, but those who really need the money do not get the grant, either because the grant application did not meet the standard criteria or those giving the grant are not paying attention to the needs of minority populations or institutions. The priority here is to be involved in grants and hire qualified faculty to spearhead and mentor the junior faculty on EBP research process.
- Lack of support from the administration. The administrator attitude, coupled with limited resources, might not deem it necessary to change from the old way of doing things. Also, the administration may hire information specialists who implement the software application without the input of the end-users: nurses.
- Knowledge deficit relating to EBP process. Some nurses do not know how or where to look for information. They would rather ask their seniors or the doctor than look for the information themselves. Many nurses have limited knowledge of research because they are not exposed to research at the beginning of their career, unlike other healthcare workers such as pharmacy and medical students.

These reasons drove the author to ensure that her RN-to-BSN online students are exposed to a capstones via research methods before graduation. Hence, selection of a topic and identification of the scholarly articles are introduced in the summer's role transition class, presiding in the first semester, in which nursing research and informatics and technology are being introduced. At this juncture, the students synthesize their review, at which time an abstract is developed. The poster is submitted in the fall semester to a conference and if accepted the students in the leadership class would then develop a poster for presentation at the conference. Figure 9.1 shows examples of poster presentations by students on supervision.

In conclusion, many consumers turn to Internet for their health-related information. There is a surge of information on the Internet, but not all information on the Web is from reliable source. For the nurse to assist patients obtain the right information and use

TABLE 9.2 Articles Retrieved Through Online Search Engines on Myocardial Infarction (2010–2015)

AUTHOR/TITLE	SAMPLE SIZE	OBJECTIVES	METHOD AND DESIGN	SUBJECTS SETTING	OUTCOMES
Smolina, K. (2012). Determinant of the decline in mortality from AMI in England	840,175	Author/Study	Population-based study using person-linked routine hospital and mortality rate	Hospital setting	Decline in the mortality rate: 43% in men and 48% in women
Sinead Brophy et al. (2010). Population-based absolute relative survival to 1 year of people with DM following MI: A cohort study using hospital admissions data	3,371	To report trends in events and mortality rate for AMI	Cohort study of two hospitals. Statistical analysis STATA	Wales hospital and England hospital	Risks for re-infarction or death or deaths for patients with DM increases.
Yeh W. et al. (2010). Population trends in incidence and outcome of acute myocardial infarction	46,086	To assess the effects of current treatment and incidence, severity of short-term mortality of myocardial infarction in large selected population	Kaiser Permanente California database. Statistical analysis using SAS software	Hospital setting. Kaiser Permanente in North California	Decrease of mortality for all myocardial infarction patients from 10.5% to 7.8%
Smolina K., Wright L., Rayner M., & Michael G. J. (2012). Long term survival and recurrence after AMI in England 2004–2010	38,7452	To provide a comprehensive account of 7 years' prognosis in 30 days' acute myocardial infarction survival in England hospital	Data taken from 2 databases. Hospital episode statistic (HES) and mortality static. Statistical analysis done on data retrieved. Both data-sets cover all of England and include information on all hospital admissions and deaths. The HES dataset provides information on all patients admitted to hospital and whose care is funded by the NHS. The mortality data are collected by the Office for National Statistics (ONS) and include all deaths that occur in England, whether in hospital or outside	Hospital in England	Survivors of either a first or recurrent of acute myocardial infarction remained higher compared to the general population over at least 7 years, particularly in middle-age individuals

Chapter 9—Data and Evidence-Based Research in Nursing | 93

Sjoerd A., & Van R. D. (2012). Short and long term mortality after MI in patients with or without DM from 1985-2008	14,434	To study temporal trends in short- and long-term outcomes after myocardial infarction (MI), according to diabetic status	We included all 14,434 consecutive patients admitted for ST-segment elevation MI or non-ST segment elevation MI at our center between 1985 and 2008. The study patients were compared according to prevalent diabetes. Temporal trend analyses were performed by comparing decades of admission (1985-1989 vs. 1990-1999 vs. 2000-2008)	Hospital. Thoraxcenter Erasmus Medical Center, Rotterdam, The Netherlands	Temporal mortality reductions after MI between 1985 and 2008 were at least as high in patients with diabetes compared with those without diabetes. However, long-term mortality remained higher in diabetic patients. Awareness of the high-risk profile of diabetic patients is warranted and might stimulate optimal medical care and outcome
Kostus, W. J. (2011). Trends in mortality rate AMI after discharge in hospital	285,397	To assess trends in the prognosis of patients with acute myocardial infarction hospitalized in New Jersey hospitals. In recent decades, in-hospital mortality has declined markedly but the decline in longer-term mortality is less pronounced, implying that mortality after discharge has worsened	Using the myocardial infarction data acquisition system (MIDAS), data were examined of the outcomes of 285,397 patients hospitalized for a first acute myocardial infarction between 1986 and 2007	New Jersey hospitals post discharge records	Post discharge mortality rate increase. Decrease less notable in 1 year
McMams D. et al (2010). Recent trends in incidence treatment and outcomes of patients with STEMI and NSTEMI	5,383	To examine recent trends in the incidence and death rates associated with the two major types of acute myocardial infarction in residents of a large central Massachusetts metropolitan area	The review of medical records of 5,383 residents of the Worcester (MA) metropolitan area hospitalized for either ST-segment elevation acute myocardial infarction (STEMI) or non-ST-segment acute myocardial infarction (NSTEMI) between 1997 and 2005 at 11 greater Worcester medical centers	Worcester (MA) metropolitan area hospitals	Recent decreases in the magnitude of STEMI, slight increases in the incidence rates of NSTEMI, and decreases in long-term mortality in patients with STEMI and NSTEMI. AMI prevention and treatment efforts have resulted in favorable decreases in the frequency of STEMI and death rates from the major types of AMI

TABLE 9.2 Articles Retrieved Through Online Search Engines on Myocardial Infarction (2010-2015) (continued)

Takii, T. (2010). Trends in AMI incidence, and mortality over 30 years in Japan	16,238 male and 6,313 females	To explore the trends of acute myocardial infarction in Japan	Complication of 43 hospitals in Japans	43 hospitals in Japan	Decrease overall in hospital mortality from 20% to 7.8% in hospital mortality in females remains high
Ahmed, E. (2014). Mortality Trends in Patients Hospitalized with the Initial Acute Myocardial Infarction in a Middle Eastern Country over 20 Years	10,915	To define temporal trends in initial acute myocardial infarction outcomes during the past 20 decades in a Middle Eastern country	Cohort study in Qatar. Logistical regression analysis	Qatar, Middle East country hospital	Increase in hospital outcomes in patient's acute myocardial infarction
Gupta, A. (2014). Trends in acute MI in young patients differences by sex, age and race	230,684	To determine sex differences in clinical characteristics, hospitalization rates, LOS, and in-hospital mortality by age group and race among young patients with AMIs using a large national dataset of U.S. hospital discharges	National Inpatient Sample, clinical characteristics, AMI hospitalization rates, LOS, and in-hospital mortality were compared for patients with AMI across ages 30 to 54 years, dividing them into 5-year subgroups from 2001 to 2010, using survey data analysis techniques.	National inpatient samples of AMI and In-hospital mortality.	AMI hospitalization rates for young people have not declined over the past decade. Young women with AMIs have more comorbidity, longer LOS, and higher in-hospital mortality than young men, although their mortality rates are decreasing
Nauta ST, Deckers JW, Akkerhuis M, Lenzen M, Simoons ML, & Ron T. van Domburg, RT, (2011). Changes in clinical profile, treatment and mortality in patient hospitalized	14,434	To quantify the impact of implementation of treatment into clinical practice on patients with ST-segment elevation myocardial infarction	All patients admitted for STEMI or NSTEMI between 1985–2008. Study categorized into three groups hospitalized between 1985–1990, 1990–2000, and 2000–2008.	US multiple ICU admission	Substantial improvement among the acute and long term inpatients hospitalized for myocardial infarction

Yysoff Y.S. & Stnefiaris, Walters H. R. (2014). Modelling Sudden Deaths from myocardial Infarction and Stroke.	568	How the probability of sudden death from MI or stroke has changed over the period of 1981–2000	Cohort study. Statistical analysis	England population study	More improvement in sudden deaths of patients with myocardial infarction than stroke
Reikvan H. & Hagen J. P. (2011). Changes in myocardial infarction mortality.		To better understand the development of cardiovascular disease over time, we have investigated the development of MI mortality in light of the decrease in MI incidence	Data on MI mortality retrieved from the Cause of Death Registry (Statistics Norway) for the period 1969–2007 were analyzed. Mortality rates (death per 100,000 inhabitants) were calculated for the total population according to sex and the age groups 0–39 years, 10-year groups in the range 40–79 years and 80 years and higher	England	Decrease in mortality rate since 1990

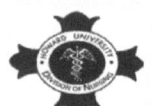
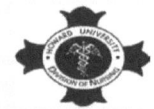

FIGURE 9.1

Source: Okunji, P. O., & Adeyemi, E. (2016). Mortality rate in myocardial infarction after treatment in myocardial infarction. In Myocardial infarction (pp. 1–5). Book Chapter, India: Avid Science.

health services, he or she must have information literacy competence. Exposing nursing students to information literacy, health literacy, and information technology skills and research early in their career helps build lasting knowledge. Nurses' educational programs must expose students to information literacy in various clinical settings. With the knowledge acquired, nurses will be ready to help consumers make sound health decisions and judgment. The knowledge acquired will equip nurses with the expertise needed to initiate evidence-based practice. Nurses need to return to school to expand their horizon in ever-expanding and demanding healthcare arena. Overall, with the introduction of Patient Care Act, electronic health records, evidence-based practice, and the emphasis in shifting to preventive and health promotion, nurses need to be well equipped to be effective, efficient, and innovative to man the ever-shifting wave of healthcare. A narrative of how research process was introduced in the author's RN-to-BSN program and a sample of a poster was shared.

STUDENTS' RESEARCH EXPERIENCE ON EVIDENCE BASE THROUGH SYSTEMIC REVIEW

TABLE 9.3 Mixed Reviewed Articles on Barriers in the Effective Management of Alcohol Addiction by Case Study, Cohort Study, and Clinical Trial

AUTHOR/DATE	ARTICLE TITLE	TYPE OF RESEARCH/ARTICLE	METHOD	LEVEL OF EVIDENCE BASE/WHY
Berl, K., Collins, M., Melson, J., Mooney, R., Muffley, C., & Wright-Glover, A. (2015)	Improving Nursing Knowledge of Alcohol Withdrawal	Case Study	Surveys were distributed to approximately 250 nurses on five medical units. Responses were obtained from 88 nurses in the pre-education survey and 92 in the post education survey. Reeducation was provided by nursing professional development specialists.	Level VI—The level of evidence is weak as surveys were used to establish the effectiveness of the implementation.
Cao, Y., Willett-Walter, C., Rimm, E., Stampfer, M., & Giovannucci, E. (2015)	Light to moderate intake of alcohol, drinking patterns, and risk of cancer: results from two prospective U.S.	Cohort Study	Using two prospective cohort studies, 88,084 women and 47,881 men participating in the Nurses' Health Study (from 1980) and Health Professionals Follow-up Study (from 1986), were followed until 2010.	Level IV—The level of evidence is moderate as evidence comes from cohort studies, which have unfiltered information.
Delker, E., Brown, Q., & Hasin, D. (2016)	Alcohol Consumption in Demographic Subpopulations: An Epidemiologic Overview	Case Study	Information was obtained from the National Epidemiologic Survey on Alcohol and Related Conditions (NESARC) and the National Survey on Drug Use and Health (NSDUH).	Level VI—The level of evidence is weak as surveys were used to establish the effectiveness of the implementation.
Dougherty, D., Lake, S., Hill-Kapturczak, N., Liang, Y., Karns, T., Mullen, J., & Roache, J. (2015).	Using Contingency Management Procedures to Reduce At-Risk Drinking in Heavy Drinkers	Clinical Trial	82 nontreatment-seeking heavy drinkers between the ages of 21 and 54 years participated in the study. Transdermal alcohol monitors were used to verify meeting contingency requirements.	Level I—The level of evidence is strong as the data is obtained from a randomized controlled trial.

TABLE 9.3 Mixed Reviewed Articles on Barriers in the Effective Management of Alcohol Addiction by Case Study, Cohort Study, and Clinical Trial *(continued)*

AUTHOR/DATE	ARTICLE TITLE	TYPE OF RESEARCH/ ARTICLE	METHOD	LEVEL OF EVIDENCE BASE/ WHY
Molina-Mula, J., González-Trujillo, A., & Simonet-Bennassar, M. (2018)	Emergency and Mental Health Nurses' Perceptions and Attitudes Towards Alcoholics	Case Study	A descriptive study was conducted in six hospitals with 167 emergency and mental health nurses.	Level VI—The level of evidence is weak as surveys were used to establish the effectiveness of the implementation.
Storholm, E., Ober, A., Hunter, S., Becker, K., Iyiewuare, P., Pham, C., & Watkins, K. (2017)	Barriers to Integrating the Continuum of Care for Opioid and Alcohol Use Disorders in Primary Care: A Qualitative Longitudinal Study	Cohort Study	Clinic administrators partook in one-on-one in-person interviews while medical and mental health providers joined in focus groups to discuss anticipated barriers and/or experienced capacity barriers to incorporating comprehensive opioid and alcohol use disorders. Data collection took place over a 3 to 4 month period at each time point.	Level IV—Level of evidence is moderate as evidence comes from cohort studies, which have unfiltered information.
Tierney, M. (2016)	Improving Nurses' Attitudes Toward Patients with Substance Use Disorders	Case Study	The author used survey that highlights stigmas and stereotypes related to substance use disorders, as well biased attitudes toward people with these problems.	Level VI—The level of evidence is weak as surveys were used to establish the effectiveness of the implementation. Surveys are prone to interviewer bias in which the interviewer might unconsciously or consciously ask questions to attempt to prove their own theory or beliefs.

Source: Armando & Okunji (2019). Manuscript on Barriers in the Effective Management of Alcohol Addiction.

TABLE 9.4 Systematic Reviewed Articles on Barriers in the Effective Management of Alcohol Addiction

AUTHOR/DATE	ARTICLE TITLE	METHOD	LEVEL OF EVIDENCE BASE/WHY
Agabio, R., Pisanu, C., Gessa, G., & Franconi, F. (2017)	Sex Differences in Alcohol Use Disorder	Reviewed sex differences in AUD by focusing on epidemiology, neurobiology, pharmacokinetic, susceptibility to medical consequences, and treatment.	Level I—The level of evidence is strong as existing literatures and data relevant to the research question were reviewed and analyzed.
Benyamina A., & Reynaud M. (2016)	Management of Alcohol Use Disorders in Ambulatory Care: Which Follow-up and for How Long?	Performed a review and analysis of the most recent literature regarding the long-term management of other chronic diseases due to the lack of official recommendations that may assist physicians in the long-term management of patients with alcohol dependence.	Level I—The level of evidence is strong as existing literatures and data relevant to the research question were reviewed and analyzed.
Dugum, M., & McCullough, A. (2015)	Diagnosis and management of alcoholic liver disease	Reviewed the diagnostic evaluation of patients with alcoholic liver disease with an emphasis on alcoholic hepatitis, discussed the current management options for these patients, and highlighted new developing therapies.	Level I—The level of evidence is strong as existing literatures and data relevant to the research question were reviewed and analyzed.
García, M., Blasco-Algora, S., & Fernández-Rodríguez, C. (2015)	Alcohol liver disease: A review of current therapeutic approaches to achieve long-term abstinence	Review and discussion of the current interventions in alcohol use disorders.	Level I—The level of evidence is strong as literatures and data relevant to the research question were reviewed and analyzed.
Leon, M., Varon, J., & Surani, S. (2016)	When a Liver Transplant Recipient Goes Back to Alcohol Abuse: Should we be More Selective?	Identified risk factors for ALD and criteria for liver transplantation by reviewing and analyzing existing literatures.	Level I—The level of evidence is strong as literatures and data relevant to the research question were reviewed and analyzed.

TABLE 9.4 Systematic Reviewed Articles on Barriers in the Effective Management of Alcohol Addiction *(Continued)*

AUTHOR/DATE	ARTICLE TITLE	METHOD	LEVEL OF EVIDENCE BASE/WHY
Maremmani, I., Cibin, M., Pani, P., Rossi, A., & Turchetti, G. (2015)	Harm Reduction as "Continuum care" in Alcohol Abuse Disorder	Used and synthesized current literatures about alcohol abuse to provide a summary about harm reduction in the treatment of alcohol abuse.	Level I—The level of evidence is strong as literatures and data relevant to the research question were reviewed and analyzed.
Quinn, A., Brolin, M., Stewart M., Evans, B., & Horgan, C. (2016)	Reducing Risky Alcohol Use: What Health Care Systems Can Do	Examined the evidence base for tools to address risky drinking and outlines policy strategies that healthcare system stakeholders may employ to address further this critical public health issue.	Level I—The level of evidence is strong as literatures and data relevant to the research question were reviewed and analyzed.
Schmidt, L. (2016)	Recent Developments in Alcohol Services Research on Access to Care	Existing literatures and data to answer questions relevant to treatment gap of alcohol use disorder.	Level I—The level of evidence is strong as existing literatures and data relevant to the research question were reviewed and analyzed.
Sudhinaraset, M., Wigglesworth, C., & Takeuchi, D. (2016)	Social and Cultural Contexts of Alcohol Use: Influences in a Social–Ecological Framework	Discussion of macrolevel factors, such as advertising and marketing, immigration and discrimination factors, and how neighborhoods, families, and peers influence alcohol use. It also describes how social and cultural contexts influence alcohol use/misuse and then explores future directions for alcohol research.	Level I—The level of evidence is strong as existing literatures and data relevant to the research question were reviewed and analyzed.

Source: Armando & Okunji (2019). Manuscript on Barriers in the Effective Management of Alcohol Addiction

Chapter 9—Data and Evidence-Based Research in Nursing | 101

TABLE 9.5 Meta-Analysis Reviewed Articles on Barriers in the Effective Management of Alcohol Addiction

AUTHOR/DATE	ARTICLE TITLE	METHOD	LEVEL OF EVIDENCE BASE/WHY
Brown, Q., Hasin, D., Keyes, K., Flink, D., Ravenell, O., & Martin, S. (2016)	Health Insurance, Alcohol and Tobacco Use Among Pregnant and Non-Pregnant Women of Reproductive Age	Explored the association between health insurance coverage and both past month alcohol use and past month tobacco use in a nationally representative sample of women age 12–44 years old.	Level 1—The level of evidence is strong as this study is a meta-analysis of randomized clinical trials.
Buzzetti, E., Kalafateli, M., Thorburn, D., Davidson, B., Thiele, M., Gluud, L., Del Giovane, C., Askgaard, G., Krag, A., Tsochatzis, E., & Gurusamy, K. (2017)	Medical Treatment of Alcohol-related Liver Disease	The Cochrane Central Register of Controlled Trials (CENTRAL), MEDLINE, Embassy, Science Citation Index Expanded, World Health Organization International Clinical Trials Registry Platform and randomized controlled trials registers until February 2017.	Level 1—The level of evidence is strong as this study is a meta-analysis of randomized clinical trials.
Foster, K., Hicks, M., Iacono, G., & McGue, M. (2015).	Gender Differences in the Structure of Risk for Alcohol Use Disorder in Adolescence and Young Adulthood	Data from a large, community sample followed longitudinally from 17 to 29 years of age, [the authors] tested for gender differences in psychosocial risk factors and consequences in adolescence and adulthood after controlling for gender differences in the base rates of AUD and psychosocial factors.	Level I—The level of evidence is strong as existing statistics, literatures and data relevant to the research question were reviewed and analyzed.
Foxcroft, D., Coombes, L., Wood, S., Allen, D., Almeida, S., & Moreira, M. (2016)	Motivational interviewing (MI) for preventing alcohol misuse in young adults is not effective enough	Identified relevant evidence from the Cochrane Central Register of Controlled Trials, MEDLINE, EMBASE and PsycINFO.	Level I—The level of evidence is strong as existing statistics, literatures and data relevant to the research question were reviewed and analyzed.
Gryczynski, J., Schwartz, R.P., O'Grady, K.E., Restivo, L., Mitchell, S., & Jaffe, G. (2016).	Understanding Patterns of High-cost Health Care use Across Different Substance User Groups	Reviewed 5 years of data from the National Survey on Drug Use and Health, the authoritative source of information on the prevalence of substance use and substance use disorders in the United States.	Level I—The level of evidence is strong as existing statistics, literatures and data relevant to the research question were reviewed and analyzed.

TABLE 9.5 Meta-Analysis Reviewed Articles on Barriers in the Effective Management of Alcohol Addiction (Continued)

AUTHOR/DATE	ARTICLE TITLE	METHOD	LEVEL OF EVIDENCE BASE/WHY
Hadland, S., Xuan, Z., Blanchette, J., Heeren, T., Swahn, M., & Naimi, T. (2015)	Alcohol Policies and Alcoholic Cirrhosis Mortality in the United States	Alcohol Policy Scale (APS), a validated assessment of policies of the 50 US states and Washington DC, to quantify the efficacy and implementation of 29 policies.	Level I—The level of evidence is strong as existing statistics, literatures and data relevant to the research question were reviewed and analyzed.
Han, B., Moore, A., Sherman, S., Keyes, K., & Palamar, J. (2017)	Demographic Trends of Binge Alcohol Use and Alcohol Use Disorders Among Older Adults in the United States, 2005–2014	Self-reported past-month binge alcohol use and AUD were estimated. Logistic regression models were used to examine correlates of binge alcohol use and AUD.	Level I—The level of evidence is strong as existing statistics, literatures and data relevant to the research question were reviewed and analyzed.
Kaner, E., Beyer, F., Muirhead, C., Campbell, F., Pienaar E., Bertholet, N.,...Burnand, B. (2018)	Effectiveness of Brief Alcohol Interventions in Primary Care Populations	Randomized controlled trials (RCTs) of brief interventions to reduce hazardous or harmful alcohol consumption in people attending general practice, emergency care or other primary care settings for reasons other than alcohol treatment.	Level I—The level of evidence is strong as existing statistics, literatures and data relevant to the research question were reviewed and analyzed.
Leasure, J., Neighbors, C., Henderson, C., & Young, C. (2015)	Exercise and Alcohol Consumption: What We Know, What We Need to Know, and Why it is Important	Relationship between physical activity and alcohol intake as exercise has been assessed as both a treatment and preventive measure.	Level I—The level of evidence is strong as existing statistics, literatures and data relevant to the research question were reviewed and analyzed.
Sacks J., Gonzales K., Bouchery, E., Tomedi, L., & Brewer, R. (2015)	2010 National and state Costs of Excessive Alcohol Consumption	From March 2012 to March 2014, the 26 cost components used to assess the cost of excessive drinking in 2006 were projected to 2010 based on incidence (e.g., change in number of alcohol-attributable deaths) and price (e.g., inflation rate in cost of medical care). The total cost, cost to government, and costs for binge drinking, underage drinking, and drinking while pregnant were estimated for the U.S. for 2010 and allocated to states.	Level I—The level of evidence is strong as existing statistics, literatures and data relevant to the research question were reviewed and analyzed.

Citation	Title	Research Design and Methods	Level of Evidence
Schuler, M., Puttaiah, S., Mojtabai, R., & Crum, R. (2015)	Perceived Barriers to Treatment for Alcohol Problems	Data from the National Epidemiologic Survey on Alcohol and Related Conditions (2001–2002) were extracted. Analyses were restricted to adults with alcohol abuse who refuses to seek treatment or dependence who reported a perceived treatment need. Latent class regression identified variables associated.	Level I—The level of evidence is strong as existing statistics, literatures and data relevant to the research question were reviewed and analyzed.
Ursic-Bedoya, J., Faure, S., Donnadieu-Rigole, H., & Pageaux, G. (2015)	Liver Transplantation for alcoholic liver disease: Lessons learned and unresolved issues	The authors utilized meta-analysis on various clinical trials.	Level I—The level of evidence is strong as existing statistics, literatures and data relevant to the research question were reviewed and analyzed.
Virtanen, M., Jokela, M., Nyberg, S., Madsen, I., Lallukka, T., & Ahola, K. (2015)	Long Working Hours and Alcohol Use: Systematic Review and Meta-Analysis of Published Studies and Unpublished Individual Participant Data	PubMed and Embase databases were used to retrieve articles across sectional and prospective studies of the association between long working hours and alcohol use. Summary estimates were obtained with random effects meta-analysis. Sources of heterogeneity were examined with meta-regression.	Level I—The level of evidence is strong as existing statistics, literatures and data relevant to the research question were reviewed and analyzed.
Xuan, Z., Blanchette, J., Nelson, T., Nguyen, T., Hadland, S., Oussayef, N., & Naimi, T. (2015)	Youth Drinking in the United States: Relationships with Alcohol Policies and Adult Drinking	Alcohol Policy Scale (APS) scores that characterized the strength of the state-level alcohol policy environments were assessed with repeated cross-sectional Youth Risk Behavior Survey data of representative samples of high school students in grades 9 to 12, from biennial years between 1999 and 2011.	Level I—The level of evidence is strong as existing statistics, literatures and data relevant to the research question were reviewed and analyzed.

Source: Armando & Okunji (2019). Manuscript on Barriers in the Effective Management of Alcohol Addiction.

TABLE 9.6 Sackett's Level I of Evidence on the Relationship between Hypertension and Inflammatory Process in African Americans with Chronic Diseases

AUTHOR/YEAR	ARTICLE TITLE	RESEARCH TYPE	BACKGROUND	METHOD	RESULTS/FUTURE RESEARCH
Gupta, Claggett, Wells, Cheng, Li, Maruthur, Selvin & Solomon (2015)	Racial Differences in Circulating Natriuretic Peptide Levels: The Atherosclerosis Risk in Communities Study	Analytical	Natriuretic peptides promote natriuresis, diuresis, and vasodilation. Experimental deficiency of natriuretic peptides leads to hypertension (HTN).	Qualitative Quantitative	African Americans have lower levels of plasma NTproBNP than White Americans, peptide levels in African Americans may contribute to the greater risk for HTN.
Hsu, Lin, Hou, (2018)	Excessive intake of fructose is associated with hypertension. Gut microbiota and their metabolites are thought to be associated with the development of hypertension.	Experimental	Consumption of daily fructose from high-fructose corn syrup and refined sugar has been on the rise over the past several decades. High-fructose (HF) diet in pregnancy has been shown to cause adverse effects on pregnancy and postnatal life. Epidemiology suggests that excessive intake of fructose is associated with numerous common diseases, including hypertension	Qualitative Quantitative	The results showed that when the rates were injected with high corn fructose, the mice became HTN.
Edmonds, Umeakunne, & Morrow (2017)	Gut Microbial Profile, Body Composition and Nutrient Intake in Obese African American Females adhering to Vegetarian and Vegan Dietary Patterns	Experimental	There is growing interest in adopting plant-based diets. There is also interest in how diet influences the gut microbiome and health.	Quantitative	Fifty percent of the women on vegetarian or vegan diet were examined for body composition (DEXA), blood pressure, nutrient intake and gut microflora. Fresh fecal samples were obtained, and major gut bacteria Revealing AA women females claiming adherence to Vegetarian Eating Parents may not be receiving adequate nutrition education on adopting a plant-based diet.

Citation	Title	Research Method	Purpose	Qualitative/Quantitative	Findings
Adnan, Nelson, Ajami, Venna, Petrosino, J.F., Bryan, & Durgan, (2017)	Alterations in the gut microbiota can elicit hypertension in rats	Experimental	Insulin resistance (IR) and impaired glucose tolerance (IGT) are the first manifestations of diet-induced metabolic alterations leading to Type 2 diabetes, while hypertension is the deadliest risk factor of cardiovascular disease.	Qualitative Quantitative	The results provide evidence that suggests that the combination of fat and sugar is potentially do more harmful than fat or sugar alone when taken in excess.
Durgan, Ganesh, Cope, Nadim, Ajami, Phillips, Petrosino, Hollister, & Bryan, (2015)	Changes in gut microbiota can elicit changes in hypertension	Experimental	Individuals suffering from obstructive sleep apnea (OSA) are at increased risk for systemic hypertension.	Qualitative Quantitative	Evidence that the gut microbiota plays a key role in the development of hypertension in the rat model of OSA with major findings. (1) In our rat model of OSA, a complicating condition, such as that associated with high-fat diet, was required to produce hypertension. (2) Gut dysbiosis, and not other factors associated with a high-fat diet, was involved in the development of OSA-induced hypertension. (3) Gut dysbiosis associated with OSA-induced hypertension involved significant decreases in bacteria involved in butyrate production and increases in bacteria involved with lactate production.
Griffin, Wang, & Stanley (2015)	Gut Microbiota Promote Angiotensin II–Induced Arterial Hypertension and Vascular Dysfunction	Experimental	The impact of gut microbiota on blood pressure and systemic.	Qualitative Quantitative	Gut microbiota facilitate vascular dysfunction driven vascular immune cell infiltration and inflammation.

TABLE 9.6 Sackett's Level I of Evidence on the Relationship between Hypertension and Inflammatory Process in African Americans with Chronic Diseases (Continued)

AUTHOR/YEAR	ARTICLE TITLE	RESEARCH TYPE	BACKGROUND	METHOD	RESULTS/FUTURE RESEARCH
Kim, Lobaton, & Raizada (2018)	Butyrate, a Microbial Metabolite, Attenuates Angiotensin II-induced Hypertension and Gut Dysbiosis.	Experimental	that hypertension (HTN) is associated with gut dysbiosis in rat models and patients with high blood pressure.	Quantitative	These observations show that gut dysbiosis and the decrease of butyrate producing bacteria are associated with Ang II-HTN.
Jandzinski, Venna, Chauhan, Graf, & McCullough, 2018	Manipulation of the Microbiome Improves Functional Recovery After Ischemic Stroke	Experiment	Circulating inflammatory markers increase with age. This pro-inflammatory milieu makes the organism less capable of coping with stressors such as stroke. Age related inflammation occurs in both the brain and peripheral tissues like the gastro-intestinal tract. There is increasing recognition that commensal bacteria in the GI tract are altered with age or with germ-free housing, affecting the brain. The change occurs most notably in the ratio of two major phyla of the microbiome, the *Firmicutes* and *Bacteroidetes*. Young age is associated with a low ratio of the two but this ratio increases with age, which has been linked to many diseases including obesity, hypertension, and diabetes which are major risk factors for stroke.	Qualitative Quantitative	We successfully reversed the microbiomes of aged organisms and gave young animals "aged" biomes. Animals with "aged" microbiomes prior to stroke had worsened functional recovery based on all behavioral tests. The "aged" biome increased mortality rates most notably in the young recipients which had over 50% mortality. Aged mice had significantly improved functional recovery as assessed by the HW test ($P < 0.05$) and NDS after reconstitution of "young" microbiome prior to stroke compared to aged control animals with the normal "aged" microbiomes.
Bryan, Nelson, & Durgan (2018)	A Role for Gut Dysbiosis in the Progression of Cerebral Small Vessel Disease	Experimental	A pathological imbalance of the gut microbiota, or dysbiosis, contributes to the inflammation that drives the progression of cerebral small vessel disease (CSVD).	Qualitative Quantitative	Although SHRSPs are a genetic model for hypertensive CSVD, the studies demonstrate that gut dysbiosis has a significant contribution to the onset of CSVD. A decrease in the abundance of healthy gut bacteria likely contributes to CSVD onset and progression.

Author	Title	Design	Method	Results
Waghulde, Cheng, Galla, Mell, Cai, Pruett-Miller, & Joe, (2018)	Attenuation of Microbiotal Dysbiosis and Hypertension in a CRISPR/Cas9 Gene Ablation Rat Model of GPER1	Experimental	G RNA CRISPR (Clustered Regularly Interspaced Short Palindromic Repeats)/Cas9 (CRISPR associated proteins) approach present with lower blood pressure, which was accompanied by altered microbiota.	Qualitative Rat Gper1 is a single exon gene with 1128 base pairs located on rat chromosome 12 (RNO12). To ensure complete gene deletion, 2 guide RNAs were designed on either end of the Gper1 gene. RNA validation performed via deletion PCR using a sense primer at the 5- end and an antisense primer at the 3- end showed a deletion PCR product of 544 bps versus wild-type PCR product of 1484 bps. This confirmed the efficiency of the dual guide RNA approach to delete Gper1. Microinjection of 10 pseudo-pregnant rats resulted in a total of 5 homozygous founders, which were used for phenotypic studies. The homozygous founders had complete deletion of Gper1, which was confirmed by DNA sequencing Homozygous founders did not express mRNA for Gper1 as demonstrated by reverse transcription PCR

Source: Pierre & Okunji (2019). Manuscript on the Relationship between Hypertension and Inflammatory Process in African Americans with Chronic Diseases.

108 | Nursing Informatics: Connecting Technology and Patient Care

TABLE 9.7 Sackett's Level II of Evidence on the Relationship between Hypertension and Inflammatory Process in African Americans with Chronic Diseases

AUTHOR/YEAR	ARTICLE TITLE	RESEARCH TYPE	BACKGROUND	METHOD	RESULTS/ FUTURE RESEARCH
Stamier, Brown, Yap, Chan, Wijeyesekera, Garicia-perez....& Elliott (2014)	Dietary and Urinary Metabonomic Factors Possibly Accounting for Higher Blood Pressure of African-Americans Compared to White Americans	Analytical	AA were compared to NHWA with high blood pressure and rates of pre-hypertension and hypertension	Questionnaire Qualitative Quantitative	Findings yield that change in AA diet did not change their blood pressure.

Source: Pierre & Okunji (2019). Manuscript on the Relationship between Hypertension and Inflammatory Process in African Americans with Chronic Diseases.

TABLE 9.8 Sackett's Level III of Evidence on the Relationship between Hypertension and Inflammatory Process in African Americans with Chronic Diseases

AUTHOR/YEAR	ARTICLE TITLE	RESEARCH TYPE	BACKGROUND	METHOD	RESULTS/FUTURE RESEARCH
Jose, & Raj (2015)	Gut microbiota in hypertension	Review study	Hypertension, which is present in about one quarter of the world's population, is responsible for about 41% of the number one cause of death, cardiovascular disease. Not included in these statistics is the effect of sodium intake on blood pressure, even though an increase or a marked decrease in sodium intake can increase blood pressure. This review deals with the interaction of gut microbiota and the kidney with genetics and epigenetics in the regulation of blood pressure and salt sensitivity.	Qualitative Quantitative	Microbiota can be controlled by many factors including diet, physical activity, genetics, and epigenetics. The influence of gut microbiota on the host may be partially explained by the generation of SCFA, including the beneficial SCFAs (acetate, butyrate, and propionate) and the non-beneficial lactate. These SCFA acting on cell surface receptors, including GPR43, GPR41, and Olfr78 regulate blood pressure. Gut microbiota can also influence the state of immunity and inflammation, cell metabolism, and proliferation that may eventually affect blood pressure.

Author	Problem	Design	Method	Findings
Walejko, Kim, Goel, Handberg, Richards, Pepine & Raizada (2018)	Black Americans have greater rates, severity, and resistance to treatment of hypertension than White Americans.	Experimental- Pilot study	Qualitative Quantitative	All four subject groups had distinct gut microbiota taxonomy by partial least squares discriminant analysis (PLS-DA). More importantly, linear discriminant analysis effect size showed marked differences in function of the microbiota of BHBP and WHBP (PLS-DA) with LDA scores <1. This included pathways for synthesis and interconversion of amino acids and inflammatory antigens. Similarly, metabolites differed (PLS-DA) with BHBP having significantly higher sulfacetaldehyde, quinolinic acid, 5-aminolevulinic acid, leucine and phenylalanine and lower 4-oxoproline and l-anserine.
Li, Zhao, Wang, Chen, Tao, Tian & Ca (2017)	Gut microbiota dysbiosis contributes to the development of hypertension	Analytical study	Qualitative Quantitative	Compared to the healthy controls, we found dramatically decreased microbial richness and diversity, Prevotella-dominated gut enterotype, distinct metagenomic composition with reduced bacteria associated with healthy status and overgrowth of bacteria such as Prevotella and Klebsiella, and disease-linked microbial function in both pre-hypertensive and hypertensive populations. Unexpectedly, the microbiome characteristic in pre-hypertension group was quite similar to that in hypertension. The metabolism changes of host with pre-hypertension or hypertension were identified to be closely linked to gut microbiome dysbiosis.

TABLE 9.8 Sackett's Level III of Evidence on the Relationship between Hypertension and Inflammatory Process in African Americans with Chronic Diseases (Continued)

AUTHOR/YEAR	ARTICLE TITLE	RESEARCH TYPE	BACKGROUND	METHOD	RESULTS/FUTURE RESEARCH
Walejko, Kim, Goel, Handberg, Richards, Pepine & Raizada (2018)	Black Americans have greater rates, severity and resistance to treatment of hypertension than White Americans.	Experimental- Pilot study	The gut microbiota and its metabolites may contribute to this. This concept was tested in a pilot study.	Qualitative Quantitative	All four subject groups had distinct gut microbiota taxonomy by partial least squares discriminant analysis (PLS-DA). More importantly, linear discriminant analysis effect size showed marked differences in function of the microbiota of BHBP and WHBP (PLS-DA) with LDA scores <1. This included pathways for synthesis and interconversion of amino acids and inflammatory antigens. Similarly, metabolites differed (PLS-DA) with BHBP having significantly higher sulfacetaldehyde, quinolinic acid, 5-aminolevulinic acid, leucine and phenylalanine and lower 4-oxoproline and l-anserine.
Tang, Kitai, & Hazen (2018)	Gut Microbiota in Cardiovascular Health and Disease	Review/ Discussions	The purpose of the current review is to highlight the complex interplay between microbiota, their metabolites and the development and progression of cardiovascular diseases. The roles of gut microbiota in normal physiology and the potential of modulating intestinal microbial inhabitants as novel therapeutic targets were discussed as well.	Qualitative Quantitative	The recent development of culture-independent techniques for microbiological analysis has uncovered the previously unappreciated complexity of The future may hold promise for targeting a microbial pathway and titrating the intervention by monitoring blood levels of the biologically active microbial derived metabolite.

Li, Zhao, Wang, Chen, Tao, Tian & Ca (2017)	Gut microbiota dysbiosis contributes to the development of hypertension	Analytical study	Recently, the potential role of gut microbiome in metabolic diseases has been revealed, especially in cardiovascular diseases. Hypertension is one of the most prevalent cardiovascular diseases worldwide, yet whether gut microbiota dysbiosis participates in the development of hypertension remains largely unknown.	Qualitative Quantitative	Compared to the healthy controls, we found dramatically decreased microbial richness and diversity, Prevotella-dominated gut enterotype, distinct metagenomic composition with reduced bacteria associated with healthy status and overgrowth of bacteria such as Prevotella and Klebsiella, and disease-linked microbial function in both pre-hypertensive and hypertensive populations. Unexpectedly, the microbiome characteristic in pre-hypertension group was quite similar to that in hypertension. The metabolism changes of host with pre-hypertension or hypertension were identified to be closely linked to gut microbiome dysbiosis.
Marchesi, Adams, Fava. Gerben, Hermes, Hirschfield, & Hart (2015)	The gut microbiota and host health: a new clinical frontier.	Review	Over the last 10–15 years, the understanding of the composition and functions of the human gut microbiota has increased exponentially. To a large extent, this has been due to new 'omic' technologies that have facilitated large-scale analysis of the genetic and metabolic profile of this microbial community, revealing it to be comparable in influence to a new organ in the body and offering the possibility of a new route for therapeutic intervention.	Qualitative Quantitative	In the past decade, interest in the human microbiome has increased considerably. A significant driver has been the realization that the commensal microorganisms that comprise the human microbiota are not simply passengers in the host, but may actually drive certain host functions as well. In sterile rodents, we see the dramatic impact that removing the microbiota has on nearly all aspects of the host's ability to function normally.

TABLE 9.8 Sackett's Level III of Evidence on the Relationship between Hypertension and Inflammatory Process in African Americans with Chronic Diseases (Continued)

AUTHOR/YEAR	ARTICLE TITLE	RESEARCH TYPE	BACKGROUND	METHOD	RESULTS/FUTURE RESEARCH
Halmos, & Suba (2017)	Physiological patterns of intestinal microbiota. The role of dysbacteriosis in obesity, insulin resistance, diabetes and metabolic syndrome	Review	The intestinal microbiota is well-known for a long time, but due to newly recognized functions, clinician's attention has turned to it again in the last decade. About 100 000 billion bacteria are present in the human intestines. The composition of bacteriota living in diverse parts of the intestinal tract is variable according to age, body weight, geological site, and diet as well. Normal bacteriota defend the organism against the penetration of harmful microorganisms and has many other functions in the gut wall integrity, innate immunity, insulin sensitivity, metabolism, and it is in cross-talk with the brain functions as well. It's a recent recognition, that intestinal microbiota has a direct effect on the brain, and the brain also influences the microbiota.	Qualitative Quantitative	Patho-mechanism is not yet cleared up. Clinicians hope, that deeper understanding of complex functions of intestinal microbiota will contribute to develop more effective therapeutic proceedings against diabetes, metabolic syndrome, and obesity.

Author	Title	Type	Findings	Method	Conclusion
Sonnenburg, & Sonnenburg (2016)	Starving our Microbial Self: The Deleterious Consequences of a Diet Deficient in Microbiota-Accessible Carbohydrates	Analytical	The gut microbiota of a healthy person may not be equivalent to a healthy microbiota. It is possible that the Western microbiota is actually dysbiosis and predisposes individuals to a variety of diseases. The asymmetric plasticity between the relatively stable human genome and the more malleable gut microbiome suggests that incompatibilities between the two could rapidly arise.	Qualitative Quantitative	The plasticity of our microbiota in response to diet was likely highly adaptive in an ancient environment. In delegating part of the digestion and calorie harvest to the gut residents, the microbial part of the biology could easily adjust to day-to-day or season-to-season variation in available food. Considering the remarkable resilience of the gut community to short-term perturbation, it is likely that microbiota adaptation is largely reversible on short time scales.
Antza, Stabouli, & Otsis (2018)	Gut microbiota in kidney disease and hypertension	Review	The human gut microbiota is being composed of more than one hundred trillion microbial cells, including aerobic and anaerobic species as well as gram-positive and negative species. Animal based evidence suggests that the change of normal gut microbiota is responsible for several clinical implications including blood pressure increase and kidney function reduction	Qualitative Quantitative	The gut microbiota dysbiosis is one of the risk factors in the progression from the advanced chronic kidney disease-CKD-to uremia, characterized by the reduction of probiotics and the increase of opportunistic pathogens including urease-related microbes, endotoxin-related microbes and toxin-related microbes, which can produce uremic toxins.
Briskey, Tucker, Johnson & Coombes (2017)	The role of the gastrointestinal tract and microbiota on uremic toxins and chronic kidney disease development	Review	It is well-established that uremic toxins are positively connected with the risk of developing chronic kidney disease and cardiovascular disease.	Qualitative Quantitative	Improvements to the microbiome, thereby potentially reducing the risk of the development of chronic kidney disease.

TABLE 9.8 Sackett's Level III of Evidence on the Relationship between Hypertension and Inflammatory Process in African Americans with Chronic Diseases (Continued)

AUTHOR/YEAR	ARTICLE TITLE	RESEARCH TYPE	BACKGROUND	METHOD	RESULTS/FUTURE RESEARCH
Koppe, & Fouque (2017)	Microbiota and prebiotics modulation of uremic toxin generation	Review	Recent data have shown that the host-intestinal microbiota interaction is intrinsically linked with overall health. Chronic kidney disease (CKD) could influence intestinal microbiota.	Qualitative	These emerging nutritional interventions may ultimately lead to a paradigm shift in the conventional focus of dietary management in CKD.
Ganesh, Nelson, Eskew, Ganesan, Ajami, Petrosino, Bryan, & Durgan (2018)	Prebiotics, Probiotics, and Acetate Supplementation Prevent Hypertension in a Model of Obstructive Sleep Apnea.	Analytical	Disruption of the gut microbiota, termed gut dysbiosis, has been described in animal models of hypertension and hypertensive patients. We have shown that gut dysbiosis plays a causal role in the development of hypertension in a rat model of obstructive sleep apnea (OSA).	Qualitative Quantitative	This indicates that probiotic and prebiotic can prevent increased SBP because of OSA but did not affect SBP in normotensive sham rats.
Pedraza-Chaverri, Sánchez-Lozada, Osorio-Alonso, Tapia, & Scholl (2017)	A New Pathogenic Concepts and Therapeutic Approaches to Oxidative Stress in Chronic Kidney Disease.	Review	In chronic kidney disease inflammatory processes and stimulation of immune cells result in overproduction of free radicals.	Qualitative	Hyperglycemia and oxidative stress play a key role in the progression of diabetic nephropathy.

Author	Title	Design	Results	Approach	Comments
Kim, Lobaton, & Raizad (2018)	Butyrate, a Microbial Metabolite, Attenuates Angiotensin II-induced Hypertension and Gut Dysbiosis.	Experimental	Gut dysbiosis was associated with an increase in Firmicutes/Bacteriodetes ratio and a decrease in butyrate-producing microbial populations.	Quantitative	These observations show that gut dysbiosis and the decrease of butyrate producing bacteria are associated with Ang II-HTN.
Taylor, & Takemiya (2017)	Hypertension Opens the Flood Gates to the Gut Microbiota. *Circulation research*.	Observation	There continues to be a rapidly evolving interest in the role of the gut microbiome in cardiovascular disease.	Quantitative	The data have provided data that, in 2 different animal models of hypertension, there is decreased of several tight junction proteins in the gut and a concomitant increase in intestinal health.
Gomez-Arango, Barrett, McIntyre, Callaway, Morrison, Nitert, & the SPRING Trial Group (2016)	Increased Systolic and Diastolic Blood Pressure Is Associated With Altered Gut Microbiota Composition and Butyrate Production in Early Pregnancy.	Review	The risk of developing preeclampsia is higher in obese pregnant women. In obesity, the gut microbiota is changed. Obesity is also associated with inflammation.	Qualitative	This study shows that in overweight and obese pregnant women at 16 weeks gestation, acquire gut.

TABLE 9.8 Sackett's Level III of Evidence on the Relationship between Hypertension and Inflammatory Process in African Americans with Chronic Diseases (Continued)

AUTHOR/YEAR	ARTICLE TITLE	RESEARCH TYPE	BACKGROUND	METHOD	RESULTS/FUTURE RESEARCH
Ramos-Romero, Hereu, Atienza, Casas, Jáuregu, Amézqueta, & Torres (2018)	Mechanistically different effects of fat and sugar on insulin resistance, hypertension, and gut microbiota in rats.	Experimental	We tested the hypothesis that gut dysbiosis contributes to hypertension in OSA. OSA was modeled in rats by inflating a tracheal balloon during the sleep cycle (10-s inflations, 60 per hour).	Qualitative Quantitative	OSA (60 apneas/hour for 8 hours during the sleep cycle) for 2 weeks had no effect on blood pressure in 10-week-old rats compared with sham rats. A. Similarly, high-fat diet alone (60% total calories from fat for 5 weeks) had no significant effect on blood pressure.
Griffin, Wang, & Stanley, 2015	Does Our Gut Microbiome Predict Cardiovascular Risk? A Review of the Evidence From Metabolomics.	Review	Millions of microbes are found in the human gut, and are collectively referred as the gut microbiota. Recent studies have estimated that the microbiota genome contains 100-fold more genes than the host genome.	Qualitative Quantitative	There is an increasing evidence that the gut microbiome has a profound effect on the systemic health of the host for a range of diseases. Obesity, type 2 diabetes mellitus, and the metabolic syndrome are some of the best characterized pathologies that have been identified as examples of these host-gut microbiome interactions, and metabolomics is increasingly being used to understand how the gut microbiome may aggravate disease processes.

Author (Year)	Title	Type	Findings	Methodology	Implications
Stecher (2015)	The Roles of Inflammation, Nutrient Availability and the Commensal Microbiota in Enteric Pathogen Infection.	Review	Gut microbiota not only plays a major role in priming and regulating mucosal and systemic immunity, but the immune system also contributes to host control over microbiota composition.	Qualitative	An increasing number of human disease conditions were linked to specific microbiota alterations.
Abais-Battad, & Mattso (2018)	The Influence of Dietary Protein on Dahl Salt-Sensitive Hypertension: a Potential Role for Gut Microbiota.	Review	Utilizing the Dahl salt-sensitive (SS) rat have demonstrated the remarkable influence of dietary protein and maternal environment on the development of hypertension and renal damage in response to high salt.	Qualitative	These studies may provide insight into the effects we have observed between diet and hypertension in Dahl SS rats and may lead to new perspectives where potential dietary interventions or microbiota manipulations could serve as plausible therapies for hypertension.

Source: Pierre & Okunji (2019). Manuscript on the Relationship between Hypertension and Inflammatory Process in African Americans with Chronic Diseases.

References

Calman N., Kitson K., & Hauser D. (2007). Using information technology to improve health quality and safety in community health centers. *Progress in Community Health Partnerships*, *1*(1), 83–88.

Earle-Foley, V. (2011). Evidence-based practice: Issues, paradigms, and future pathways. *Nursing Forum, 46*(1), 38–44

Foster, R. (2016). How the big data tools ACA, HITECH enable will improve care. *Government Health IT*. Retrieved from http://www.govhealthit.com/news/how-big-data-tools-aca-hitech-enable-will-improve-care

Gibbons M. C. (2005). A historical overview of health disparities and the potential of eHealth solutions. *Journal of Medical Internet Research,* 7(5), e50.

Gulzar, S., Khoja, S., & Sajwani, A (2013). Experience of nurses with using eHealth in Gilgit-Baltistan, Pakistan: A qualitative study in primary and secondary healthcare. *BMC Nursing,12:6*. Retrieved from https://bmcnurs.biomedcentral.com/articles/10.1186/1472-6955-12-6

Ketcham J. D, Lutfey K. E., Gerstenberger E., Link C. L., & McKinlay J. B. (2009). Physician clinical information technology and health care disparities. *Medical Care Research and Review, 66*(6), 658–681.

National Center for Education Statistics. (2015). Adulty Literacy in America. Retrieved from https://nces.ed.gov/

ODPHP (2010) National Action Plan to Improve Health Literacy. Retrieved from https://health.gov/communication/HLActionPlan/pdf/Health_Literacy_Action_Plan.pdf

Okunji, P. O., & Adeyemi, E. (2016). Mortality rate in myocardial infarction after treatment in myocardial infarction. In *Myocardial infarction* (pp. 1–5). India: Avid Science.

Olson, L.M. Library (2018). Evaluating Internet Sources, A Library Resource Guide: https://library.nmu.edu/guides/userguides/webeval.htm

Saba, V., & McCormick, K. (2011). *Essentials of nursing informatics.* (5th ed.). New York, NY: McGraw-Hill.

Sewell, J., & Thede, L. (2013). *Informatics and nursing opportunities and challenges.* (4th ed). Philadelphia, PA: Lippincott Williams & Wilkins.

Shipman, J. P., Kurtz-Rossi, S., & Funk, C. J. (2009). The health information literacy research project. *Journal of the Medical Library Association,* 97(4), 293–301. doi:10.3163/1536-5050.97.4.014

U.S. Department of Health and Human Services (2000). Freedom of Information Act. *Healthy people (2020).* Retrieved from https://www.healthypeople.gov/

United States National Library of Medicine (2016). NLM's university-based biomedical informatics research training programs. Retrieved from https://www.nlm.nih.gov/ep/GrantTrainInstitute.html.

United States Department of Health and Human Services (2000). *Healthy People 2010.* Washington, DC: U.S. Government Printing Office. Originally developed for Ratzan SC, Parker RM. 2000. Introduction. In *National Library of Medicine Current Bibliographies in Medicine: Health Literacy.* Selden CR, Zorn M, Ratzan SC, Parker RM, Editors. NLM Pub. No. CBM 2000-1. Bethesda, MD: National Institutes of Health, U.S. Department of Health and Human Services.

Figure Credits

Table 9.1 Sources: https://www.ncbi.nlm.nih.gov/pubmed/20923995, https://www.ncbi.nlm.nih.gov/pubmed/21187184, https://www.ncbi.nlm.nih.gov/pubmed/19942783, https://www.ncbi.nlm.nih.gov/pubmed/25060366, https://www.ncbi.nlm.nih.gov/pubmed/21383800

Fig. 9.1: Copyright © Okunji, P. O., Adeyemi, E. (CC by 4.0) at http://www.avidscience.com/wp-content/uploads/2016/05/RAMI-16-01_April-11-2016.pdf.

UNIT IV

CHAPTER 10

E-Health: Disease Prevention and Management

CHAPTER HIGHLIGHTS

This chapter discusses the following:

- How healthcare is becoming personalized and mobile health (mHealth) could be designed to offer personal toolkits for predictive, participatory, and preventative care
- How access to information is becoming so easy and patients are taking responsibility for their own health, hence the development of consumer informatics, a subspecialty in healthcare informatics
- How Telehealth and Telemedicine have been used in the past to refer patients to health services, delivered using electronic or telecommunication devices to assess patients at a distance.
- How easy availability and the push for a more cost-effective healthcare delivery system is a desire of most consumers and has led to the advent of health portals, which is mainly government sponsored

HEALTHCARE, LIKE OTHER industries, is becoming personalized. mHealth could be designed to offer personal toolkits for predictive, participatory, and preventative care. Of the 74% who used the Internet in 2008, 80% used online health information, which translates to 59% of all adults in the United States. (Breuer & Meier, 2012). Various studies have reported that social media usage and effectiveness for individuals worldwide has increased over the years, and social networking now accounts for 22% of all time spent online in the United States. (Jencks, Williams, & Coleman, 2009). A total of 234 million people aged 13 and older in the United States used mobile devices in 2008 (Jencks et al., 2009), and this trend has increased since that time. Internet page views occurred most frequently at one of the top social networking sites in December 2009, up from 13.8% a year before (Kocher & Adashi, 2011). It is reported that the number of social media users age 65 and older increased by approximately 100% throughout 2010, so that one in four people in that age group now belong to a social networking site. Technology is being used as a means of improving access to care, while reducing costs of transportation and increasing convenience to patients in accessing care (Krumholz et al., 2011). Technology encompasses preventive, promotive, and curative aspects.

Diabetes affects 26 million people in the United States, of which 7 million are undiagnosed (Centers for Disease Control and Prevention, 2011). According to the Center for Disease Control and Prevention (2011), between 1980 through 2011 the number of individuals with diabetes has tripled from 5.6 million to 20.9 million. Nowhere has this epidemic been more noticeable than in the hospital setting (Fowler, 2009). Patients hospitalized with diabetes make up approximately 12 to 25% of hospital admissions (Centers for Disease Control and Prevention, 2011). The rate of diabetes hospitalizations will continue to escalate if innovative preventive measures are not put in place. Studies have shown that the contributing variables to this rise include higher prevalence of obesity, changes in diagnostic criteria, a growing elderly population, and growth in minority populations in whom the prevalence and incidence of diabetes are increasing (Kamaruddin, Quinton, & Leech, 2008). The actual national cost is estimated to be over $174 billion when other burdens, such as the social cost of intangibles like pain and suffering, care provided by non-paid caregivers, excess medical costs associated with undiagnosed diabetes, and diabetes-attributed costs for healthcare expenditures categories are included (Kamaruddin, Quinton, & Leech, 2008). It is estimated that by 2025 this number of diabetic patients will rise to at least 30 million (Knowles et al., 2002). Diabetes is common amongst hospitalized patients with a prevalence rate of about 30% (Breuer & Meier, 2012).

Studies have shown that readmission following an inpatient hospitalization is fairly common, and costly and frequent hospital readmissions and unexplained variances may indicate poor quality in healthcare, transitions of care, and outpatient management following discharge (Jencks, Williams, & Coleman, 2009). However, while some readmissions may be inevitable, reducing hospital readmissions has been a critical variable of several recent government efforts to improve quality and reduce costs in the federal insurance companies, such as the Medicare program (Kocher & Adashi, 2011). MI has been identified as a common reason for Medicare hospitalizations and has been found to have a relatively high readmission rate (Krumholz et al., 2011). Six hundred and thirty-three inpatient MI hospital stays were reported in the United States in 2009 Health Care Utilization Project Network (HCUPnet, 2009). According to the 2008 National Healthcare Disparity Report, MI mortality in 2005 was 652,091, ranking first while diabetes ranked sixth with a mortality rate of 75,119 and total cost of $174 billion, with $116 billion in direct medical costs. The total cost for cardiovascular diseases in 2008 was $448.5 billion, with a direct medical cost of $296.4 billion (National Healthcare Disparities Report, 2009). The total estimated cost of diagnosed diabetes in 2012 is $245 billion, including $176 billion in direct medical costs and $69 billion in reduced productivity (American Diabetes Association, 2012). Up to now, no studies have focused on 30-day readmission rates by patients and hospital characteristics on diabetic MI (Breuer & Meier, 2014). Hence, it was recommended that examining characteristics that explain differences in readmission rates can help to identify opportunities for targeted interventions for hospital patients at risk for readmission, such as patients hospitalized for MI (Stranges, Barrett, Wier, & Andrews, 2012).

E-HEALTH

E-health is defined as "the utilization of information, and communication technologies to support health and health related fields, such as health surveillance, healthcare services, health literature, health education and research" (Gulzar, Khoja, & Sajwani, 2013).

The goal is to improve the consumer decision-making processes and health outcomes with electronic information and communication (American Medical Information Technology Association, 2010). In a research study carried out in Pakistan by Gulzar and colleagues (2013), it was found that e-health was beneficial to healthcare providers by improving their professional development and patient outcome; it saved time and provided communication and learning opportunities, as well as communication between healthcare providers at different levels, preventing professional isolation for providers in remote areas.

In the past, patients were not as knowledgeable as the healthcare providers, which developed a culture, which is paternalistic. The expectation is that the patient accepts what was prescribed without any consideration of the cost. Patients were labeled as noncompliant if they did not comply. The question to be asked is why is a consumer who is able to buy care, a computer, and other high-priced items cannot do the same for healthcare. The answer is that they have not been allowed to do so. The Leapfrog Group is comprised of large corporations who came together and studied how they could influence the quality and affordability of healthcare and give consumers more control over how to spend their money. This has been on the increase; it has been made possible with the Internet and World Wide Web. Today, consumers can learn and search for information about diseases, which they did not have access to before. The face of the healthcare industry is permanently changing to one of consumerism. There is easy access to information, and patients are taking responsibility for their own health, hence the development of consumer informatics, a subspecialty in healthcare informatics.

TELEHEALTH

Standard nursing practice involves using one's senses and instinct for the assessment and care of a patient. Nurses were taught to use the sense of touch to answer questions such as (a) Is their skin warm, cold and clammy? (b) Is the patient's skin color normal? (c) Is the patient alert to a person, place, and time? How do nurses assimilate these common nursing practices into the current state of healthcare technology such as telehealth and telemedicine? (Beck, 2005). The use of information technology has increased in different parts of the world, hence the use of words such as telenursing, telehealth, telehomecare, and telepresence. Telehealth nursing is used when delivering care remotely is needed, which improves efficiency and access to healthcare. It is usually practiced in the home, healthcare clinics, doctor's offices, prisons, hospitals, telehealth nursing call centers, and mobile units.

Telehealth has the ability to improve care as well as reduce travel time and distance. One of the advantages of telehealth is improvement in patient outcomes due to central data storage. As a result of this centralized storage, there is improved coordination of care. It is a powerful health tool for managing patients with chronic disease. Through telehomecare, patient's vital signs, and cardiac rhythm, blood glucose and weight can be sent and stored in a patient's record.

Many nurses may have practiced telehealth nursing without knowing it. According to Westra (2012), any nurse who has spoken with a patient over the phone has practiced telehealth nursing. A 2005 International Telenursing Survey with 719 telehealth full- and part-time nurses (registered nurses, and advanced practice nurses) showed that of 49 states (Delaware was not represented) and 36 countries around the world (USA (68%), Canada (10%), Australia (5%), United Kingdom (4%), Norway (3.5%), New Zealand (1.1%), Sweden (1%), Iran (0.6%), and Finland (0.6%), three countries had three telehealth nurses, seven countries had two telehealth nurses, and 17 countries had one telehealth nurse (Westra, 2012).

TELENURSING

Telenursing is defined as "the use of telemedicine technology to deliver nursing care and conduct nursing practice" (Beck, 2005).

> Over the past several years, technological innovations and Internet-based communication have occurred at a rapid and continually evolving rate. Internet based services can be provided using several technological platforms, including Web sites, videoconferencing applications, and hand held devices. Advantages of these technologies include their ease of access and increasingly widespread use. Remote treatments allow individuals who are unable or unwilling to seek in-person treatment to obtain services while located at the preferred places such as home, work place, or even hotel room if travelling. (Yuen, Goetter, Herbert, & Forman, 2011, p. 1)

Telehealth and telemedicine have been used in the past to refer to health services delivered using electronic or telecommunication device to patients at a distance. According to American Telemedicine Association (ATA), telemedicine refers to the electronic exchange of patient information between two sites for improving the patient's health status and telehealth; a broader term extends beyond the delivery of clinical services (American Telemedicine Association, 2010). The United Kingdom is encouraging healthcare care providers to adopt telehealth programs as part of their care strategy for patients with long-term conditions.

> "The current era of healthcare reform is driving a shift in priorities and pressures for delivery of high-quality healthcare. With a surge in the need to efficiently meet patient care demands, and to accommodate the ever-evolving sophistication and modernization of information and communication technologies (ICT), it is an opportune time for innovative care delivery by telehealth. Telehealth can increase access to primary and specialty care, and ensure high quality care at lower cost." (Fathi, Modin & Scott, 2017, p. 1).

It is very important to consider some of the safety issues before choosing the telehealth method in providing care to the patient. Some of the safety problems to consider as a telehealth nurse include assessing the patient's ability and health status, knowing the equipment, evaluating reliability, infection control, information safety, and compliance with nursing judgment.

TELEHEALTH METHODS

Some of the telehealth methods include real time and telephone based and are sometimes limited to education and counseling and web-consults (two-way audio and video), with or without peripheral devices, store-and-forward images, and audio and video combination.

The two main uses in technology are store and forward (S&F) or two communications and real-time health. In S&F technology, a digital camera, scanner, or other piece of technology (e.g., an X-ray machine) that generates electronic images to capture a still image electronically and send that image to a specialist for interpretation (American Telemedicine Association, 2010). Other departments in the hospital such as radiology, dermatology, pathology, and wound care specialties also use this type of technology. It also includes nonsynchronous transmission of clinical data, which may include the results of an electrocardiogram, magnetic resonance imaging, blood glucose levels may be sent to two different sites. This type of communication is usually between two healthcare providers. This type of technology has made it possible for medicine to be practiced in remote areas. For example, S&F is used when a radiologist is located at a different site from where the X-ray was taken and still reads the X-ray. This method is frequently used in healthcare (Sewell & Thede, 2013).

IN REAL-TIME TELEHEALTH

It is possible for the patient and provider to interact at the same time by using interactive video/television. One of the devices that permits two-way communication is video conferencing, which requires at least a T1 line or a line integrated to a digital network, which not only connects sites, but also extends to the rooms where both the patient and consultant are located. Real-time telehealth uses special equipment that can transmit information to a clinician at a different location. These instruments include ear-nose-throat scopes, cameras used for skin observations, and special stethoscopes. These instruments may be used in real time or in S&F mode. One of the advantages of this technology is that a surgeon, with the help of a robot, virtual reality, special gloves, and appropriate audio/video technology, may be able to perform surgery through a remote site. This type of procedure uses telepresence. Telepresence is the use of technology to provide the appearance of a person's presence, although he or she is located at a remote site. (Sewell & Thede, 2013). Equipment needed includes phone lines, the Internet, a phone or computer with or without a camera, cell phones, a lifeline, sensor technology, and peripheral devices (Westra, 2012).

TELEHOMECARE

Some of the means through which telehealth can be delivered is through telehomecare, portable monitoring devices, wearable monitoring garments, and peripheral devices. One of the greatest advantages of this type of care is that healthcare and monitoring is provided at the convenience of the patient's home, rather than the provider's work setting. Telehealth can be used in an interactive way by also tracking patients. It is cost saving to payers due to a reduction in utilization by chronic patients and a reduction in hospital stays. If admission and hospital stays are reduced, less is needed by agencies that use telehealth. Home health agencies that utilize telehealth have an average patient ratio to registered nurse of 15:1, while the agencies without telehealthcare ratio is 11:1 (Peck, 2005). Elderly care use of telehealth strategies include transitional care for heart failure, palliative care, chronic disease, mental health management and behavioral health, home based primary care for frail older adults, remote monitoring, and supports for family caregivers (Quinn, O'Brien, and Springan, 2018).

> Older adults with complex care needs want to live as independently as they can for as long as they can, and limit stress on family caregivers. Telehealth strategies offer the potential to improve access to care and the quality of care, while reducing strain on family caregivers. For healthcare systems, home telehealth may help address the challenge of rising costs. Though limited today, home telehealth is likely to be implemented more widely as policy makers reduce regulatory barriers and providers focus on improving telehealth strategies to meet the needs of families. (Quinn, O'Brien, and Springan, 2018, p. 1)

Some of the portable monitoring devices have similarities. Many of the devices use a touch screen, text, and audio for patient health assessment; ask questions ("On a scale of 0–10 … ?"; "Yes or no …"); and may also be programmed to include branching questions, which result in patient education. The devices include the following:

- Pill dispensers/reminders are devices used in telehomecare. They may include an auditory reminder to alert the patient to take his or her medication. It may also remind patients to take the medication with food or take their insulin; if the medications are not taken as scheduled, the caregiver may be notified by telephone; if the caregiver does not answer, the call will go to the support center.
- A wearable monitoring garment is a fascinating concept that makes it possible for symptoms to be identified early before problems develop. This concept of smart underwear has sensors printed on the waistband for monitoring. The underwear senses, makes diagnoses, and dispenses appropriate medications. This technology is being developed for warriors who are injured in battle and for others who are sick.
- Peripheral devices may be used and include blood pressure machines, scales, glucose monitoring, EKG/cardiac monitoring, otoscopes and pedometers (Westra, 2012). Peripheral devices such as electroencephalogram and electrocardiography, blood oxygen saturation, and blood pressure measures. Research has shown that wearable devices have the ability to detect symptoms and treat depression, epilepsy, Parkinson's disease, and hypothermia.

There is also a shirt for cardiac and respiration monitoring with blood pressure cuff and weight scale that is Bluetooth enabled for data transmission. Various studies have been conducted in telehomecare. In one of the studies conducted by the Veteran Administration, one group was monitored weekly and their wounds were photographed and then mailed it to the coordinator for evaluation and follow up. The second group reported, using a telehealth monitoring device, reported disease management data daily to the care coordinator. The group that used telehomecare to report had improved outcomes over the group that was monitored weekly.

Telehomecare can also be used in the management of chronic patients such as those with heart failure. This technology is used worldwide and has led to a reduction in hospitalization rates and services provided. A medical center in Atlanta, Georgia, reported that telehomecare monitoring heart failure patient readmission was 75% lower than that for patients not in the program (Sewell & Thede, 2013).

TELEMENTAL HEALTH

It is important to note that psychologists have found a way to treat a wide range of disorders by developing innovative treatments. Unfortunately, many patients with such problems do not have access to or are undertreated for the cure they desperately need (Yuen et al., 2011; Grant et al., 2006). Mental healthcare specialists are sometimes hard to find, especially in the rural areas of the United States. Sometimes people with mental problems have difficulty accessing healthcare due to organizational problems such as limited transportation, limited physicians, and disability and scheduling difficulties. Often times, some of the patients are reluctant to seek care because of psychological issues such as anxiety and fear of leaving home, traveling, and interacting with unfamiliar people. Internet-based technology can be used to provide care in rural areas, which traditionally have few options for specialists. In Maine, it was reported that some of the island had many barriers, and they depend on seafood for their livelihood. Oftentimes, people in these areas do not travel because of loss of income and inconvenience. To address their healthcare problems, a company named Sunbeam Island services started providing clinic visits by using a ship staffed by nurses and equipped with two-way teleconference equipment. The ship has the ability to connect to seven hubs on the mainland. This visit is conducted twice per month. The residents visit the clinic where nurses can make initial assessments (Sewell & Thede, 2013).

E-INTENSIVE CARE UNITS

The monitoring of critical care patients is not new to research. The use of telepresence in the intensive care unit brought a new meaning to monitoring patients in the critical care units. The mortality rate of ICU patients decreased 10–20% (Leapfrog Group, 2010).

ROBOTICS: RP-7 ROBOT

R-P means remote presence. It is one of the means through which telepresence helps the intensivists provide care for patients. It stands at about 5 feet 6 inches, with a large flat-screen monitor, small camera and zoom features, and a couple of antennas. It has the ability to receive and transmit data through a wireless network. The robot rolls on three spheres with a built-in infrared sensing device to help guide it around obstacles.

The remote intensivist expert controls the robot with a joystick. This technology can be used with either a laptop or a desktop computer (Robotics Today, 2018).

TELETRAUMA CARE

The advancement in technology has made it possible for rural hospitals to provide trauma care and get reimbursements for these services. Tele-trauma can also be used to obtain second opinions from trauma care experts.

DISASTER HEALTH

During a major disaster (Hurricane Katrina) in the Gulf States, a Katrina website was up and running and was used to facilitate communication and assist victims in accessing electronic prescription medication records.

Telehealth has presented opportunities for nurses to develop autonomy in their practice. It has presented nurses the opportunity to develop nurse-led service and telehealth service with minimum physician or consultant input, except in exceptional circumstances (Anguita, 2012). It is possible for one nurse to manage many patients and telehealth has made this possible.

Mercy Health Center in Laredo Texas was a good example of how implementing a telehealth disease management program can reduce cost from utilization while improving outcomes and patient satisfaction. After [a] one-year decrease, reductions in overall utilization and charges, as well as improvements in quality were demonstrated. Charge reductions in diabetes related care for the disease management program were $747 per patient year, compared with standard care (Peck, 2005, p. 339–343, https://journals.lww.com/naqjournal/Citation/2005/10000/Changing_the_Face_of_Standard_Nursing_Practice.8.aspx).

TELEHEALTH ISSUES

Some of the main issues in implementing telehealth are as follows:

- Reimbursement: One of the questions often asked is who will pay for telehealth. According to Peck, 2005, "There are currently no consistent, comprehensive reimbursement guidelines. Though the federal government has passed statutes to promote telehealth, the provisions have fallen short of incentives from physicians and healthcare organizations to implement it. For telehealth to be successful, reimbursement must be a joint effort between the state, federal government and private payers" (Peck, 2005, pp. 339–343, https://insights.ovid.com/crossref?an=00006216-200510000-00008)
- Technical: Patient safety is of utmost concern with development and usage of this new technology. Simply, telehealth will not function without electronic health records. Transmitting healthcare records is only one part of the problem; making data available when it is needed by the provider is bigger problem. Different data standards have different technological implications when it comes to data

translation and the sharing of medical information. Other problems include slow deployment of medical technology, potential fraud and abuse, and privacy issues.
- Legislation and policy: Telehealth raises a lot of policy issues in the area of licensure. This problem is primarily because professional nursing associations, unions, state regulatory boards, and Congress have not come to an agreement on multistate licensure, and the critical question is how it will be implemented.

According to research, people were satisfied with being cared for in the privacy of their homes. Technology and telehealth has evolved since the publication of telehealth between 2001 and 2007, which revealed significant and positive outcomes (Sewell & Thede, 2013).

IMPACT OF TELEHEALTH

The impact of telehealth is phenomenal. Studies have shown that it is safe and effective when compared to conventional treatments. Telehealth can be used in student clinical experience in an effort to enhance their learning. This can be achieved by providing health education and monitoring and evaluating lifestyles. Valuable information and experience can be gathered through this method. The easy availability and the push for a more cost-effective healthcare delivery system is a desire of most consumers. It has led to the advent of health portals, which is mainly government sponsored. The patient portal offers one-way communication, which may be specific to one patient. Some examples include sending diabetic patients reminders about making an appointment for a foot check or alerting patients about abnormally high cholesterol results with a link to a video about video control. Some portals allow the patient to upload blood glucose results and then provide a feedback on glucose control. This type of personalization was made possible through telehealth. One of the biggest criticisms of advanced technology is the digital divide or the information inequality/information gap. In some developing countries, the ability to tap into these resources may not be available. The emphasis now is on a participatory approach than on the paternalistic approach.

There are challenges and disadvantages with e-health. These challenges include increased workload and dealing with technology-related problems such as installation, picture quality, and sound quality. One of the biggest concerns is patients' privacy and security.

CYBERCHONDRIACS

Consumer searches have led to the new term "cyberchondriacs." This term basically refers to a person who has concerns about health and searches for health information on the Web. According to researchers at Harris Interactive, many people have concerns regarding searching information on the Web because they believe that healthcare provider relationships will erode. But this assertion was not true. The 2002 survey reported that 30% of the U.S online population, 23% of the population in France, 33% in Germany, and 17% in Japan discovered that online information influenced the discussions with their healthcare providers. They also found that that this information affected their understanding of healthcare problems and overall improved their health management (Sewell & Thede, 2013).

INTERNET PHARMACIES

Internet pharmacies will also be affected by increased use of advanced technology. Most online pharmacies require a prescription and have a pharmacy portal that allows consumers to renew and order prescriptions online. The portal includes services such as patient education on drugs and an e-mail or text message when a prescription is ready. The high cost of drugs has led to a search for less expensive alternatives on the Web. This created a problem whereby pharmacies allow consumers to purchase medications without consultation or prescription from a healthcare provider. More importantly, they may sell counterfeit or out-of-date medication, provide a wrong dosage, or sell a medication that has the potential for creating a drug reaction and includes no warning to buyer's possible side effects or instructions for the appropriate method of taking the medication. Even though, in 2010, various search engines such as Google, Bing, and Yahoo agreed to a policy to allow only verified Internet pharmacy practice sites to advertise on their websites; pharmacies that are not verified still show up on Web searches (Sewell & Thede, 2013).

References

American Academy of Ambulatory Nursing (2018). *Telehealth nursing practice.* Retrieved from https://www.aaacn.org/community/telehealth-nursing-practice-sig

American Diabetes Association. (2012). Economic costs of diabetes in the U.S. in 2012. *Diabetes Care, 36*(4), 1033–1046. Retrieved from http://care.diabetesjournals.org/content/36/4/1033.full

Anguita, M. (2012). Opportunities for nurse led telehealth and telecare. *Nurse Prescribing*, 10(1), 6–8.

Beck, A. (2005). Changing the face of standard nursing practice through telehealth and telenursing. N*ursing Administration* Quarterly, 29:4. https://journals.lww.com/naqjournal/Citation/2005/10000/Changing_the_Face_of_Standard_Nursing_Practice.8.aspx

Breuer, T. G., & Meier J. J. (2012). Inpatient treatment of type 2 diabetes. Dtsch Arztebl International, *109*(26), 466–74. Retrieved from https://www.aerzteblatt.de/int/archive/article/127211/Inpatient-treatment-of-type-2-diabetes

Centers for Disease Control and Prevention (2011). National diabetes fact sheet: National estimates and general information on diabetes and pre-diabetes in the United States. Atlanta, GA: U.S. Department of Health and Human Services. Retrieved from https://www.cdc.gov/diabetes/pubs/pdf/ndfs_2011.pdf

Fathi, J. T., Modin, H.E., Scott, J.D., (May 31, 2017). "Nurses Advancing Telehealth Services in the Era of Healthcare Reform" *OJIN: The Online Journal of Issues in Nursing* Vol. 22, No. 2, Manuscript DOI: 10.3912/OJIN.Vol22No02Man02

Fowler, M. J. (2009). Inpatient diabetes management. *Clinical Diabetes, 27,* 119–122.

Grant, K. E., Compas, B. E., Thurm, A. E., McMahon, S. D., Gipson, P. Y., Campbell, A. J., ... & Westerholm, R. I. (2006). Stressors and child and adolescent psychopathology: Evidence of moderating and mediating effects. *Clinical Psychology Review 26*(3), 257–283.

Gulzar, S., Khoja, S., & Sajwani, A. (2013). Experience of nurses with nurses with using eHealth in Gilgit-Baltistan, Pakistan: A qualitative study in primary and secondary healthcare. *Biomed Central Nursing*, 12:6. https://bmcnurs.biomedcentral.com/articles/10.1186/1472-6955-12-6

HCUPnet (2009). *Healthcare Cost and Utilization Project (HCUP)*. Retrieved from http://hcupnet.ahrq.gov

Jencks, S. F., Williams, M. V., & Coleman, E. A. (2009). Rehospitalizations among patients in the Medicare Fee-for-Service program. *New England Journal of Medicine 360*, 1418–1428.

Kamaruddin, M. S., Quinton, R., & Leech, N. (2008). Standards of medical care in diabetes—First Do No Harm. Inpatient diabetes management (RQ) final.doc. Retrieved from https://www.researchgate.net/publication/234128632_Inpatient_diabetes_care_first_do_no_harm

Knowles, W. C., Barrett-Connor, E., Fowler, S. E., Hamman, R. F., Lachin, J. M., & Walker, E. A. (2002). Reduction in the incidence of type 2 diabetes with lifestyle intervention or metformin. *New England Journal of Medicine 346*, 93–403.

Kocher, R. P., & Adashi, E. Y. (2011). Hospital readmissions and the Affordable Care Act. Paying for coordinated quality care. *Journal of American Medical Association, 306*(16), 1794–1795.

Krumholz, H. M., Lin, Z., Drye, E. E., Desai, M. M., Han, L. F., Rapp, M. T., ... & S. L. (2011). An administrative claims measure suitable for profiling hospital performance based on 30-day all-cause readmission rates among patients with acute myocardial infarction. *Circulation Cardiovascular Quality and Outcomes, 4*(2), 243–52.

Leapfrog Group. (2010). NQF Safe Practices for Better Healthcare 2010 About us. Retrieved from http://www.leapfroggroup.org/about

National Healthcare Disparities Report. (2009). Summary. *Agency for Healthcare Research and Quality*. Retrieved from http://www.ahrq.gov/qual/nhdr03/nhdrsum03.htm

Peck, A. (2005). Changing the face of standard nursing practice through telehealth and telenursing. *Nursing Administration Quarterly, 29*(4), 339–343.

Robotics Today. (2018). *RP-7*. Retrieved from https://www.roboticstoday.com/robots/rp-7-description

Sewell, J. & Thede, S. (2013). *Informatics and nursing* (4th ed.). Philadelphia, PA. Lippincott Williams & Wilkins.

Stranges, E., Barrett, M., Wier, L., & Andrews, R. (2012). Readmissions for heart attack (Statistical Brief No. 140). *Healthcare Cost and Utilization Process*. Retrieved from http://www.ncbi.nlm.nih.gov/books/NBK109195/

Westra, B. (2012). Telenursing and Remote Access Telehealth. *Nursing informatics—deep dive*, Integrating Quality, Safety and Education (QSEN) Strategies into Nursing Competences. Retrieved from https://www.google.com/search?q=Westra,+B.+(2012).+Nursing+informatics%E2%80%94deep+dive.+Retrieved+from&tbm=isch&tbo=u&source=univ&sa=X&ved=2ahUKEwi-mNK_krLfAhXtY98KHREoDXwQsAR6BAgFEAE&biw=866&bih=684

Yuen, E., Goetter, E. & Herbert, H, & Forman, E. M. (2011). Challenges and opportunities in Internet mediated telemental health. *American Psychological Association, 43*(1), 1–8.

Quinn W. V., O'Brien E., and Springan G. (2018). Using Telehealth to Improve Home-Based Care for Older Adults and Family Caregivers. AARP Real Possibilities. *Public Health Institute*. Retrieved from https://www.aarp.org/content/dam/aarp/ppi/2018/05/using-telehealth-to-improve-home-based-care-for-older-adults-and-family-caregivers.pdf

CHAPTER 11

Health Information Systems and Patient Safety

CHAPTER HIGHLIGHTS

This chapter discusses the following:

- How electronic documentation (EMR and EHR) has promised error-free data and information could be used as evidence that the nursing intervention occurred
- How strong passwords are used to secure the confidential information of the organization and the information that is not in regular use of the organization
- How remote access to every bit of information about a patient in one centralized place is the most useful element of electronic medical records for nurses
- How secured servers would be safe havens for the preservation and protection of patients' clinical information and their hospitals via rigorous system planning and execution

THE ROLE OF electronic documentation using standardized terminologies in informing evidence-based nursing care is amazing. The nursing practice involves the collection, evaluation, storage and retrieval of information gathered from an individual, family, or community (Schwirian, 2013). The primary objective of electronic documentation is to collect information required to identify the problems of patients and symptoms that are sensitive to the nursing practice. Nursing assessment, therefore, provides an evidence base for making communications and referrals to other disciplines. The database of nursing assessment avails the foundation of care planning and the basis for evaluating the status of the patients. Accurate, complete, and ubiquitous patient assessment data and information lead to effective care and automation of data (Saba & Taylor, 2007). Electronic documentation promises error-free data and information that can be used as evidence that the nursing intervention occurred.

Healthcare providers need to determine the best approaches for incorporating the elements of nursing into electronic health records. Electronic documentation ensures long-term preservation and storage of records, which promotes evidence-based nursing care. An accurate nursing database is a critical element in the nursing profession because it ensures effective communication and easy problem identification, making intervention plans and evaluation of patient progress through the recovery process (Busch, 2008). This is because accurate databases avail up-to-date information that is used by nurses in their professional practice. A detailed model of assessment data maintains the quality of data, consistency in documentation, and support in evidence-based planning in the nursing practice. Data stored is used for supporting the evidence that the medical intervention took place and the nurse who is responsible for the alleged nursing process. Standardized nursing terminologies and guidelines support the diagnoses, interventions, and outcomes of the nursing process through availing evidence of prior treatments by the standardized nursing terminologies, a national survey of nurses' experiences and attitudes (Thede & Schwiran, 2011).

Electronic documentation enables transmission of data through a codified format. Standardized content alone is not sufficient to support evidence-based nursing practice. Medical practitioners capture atomic-level data that reflects actual patient status (Saba & Taylor, 2007). This data needs to be transferred through a structured and codified format to make it possible for easy storage, retrieval, and analysis in both the present and the future. International Classification for Nursing Practice (ICNP) provides a foundation for capturing atomic level data. ICNP data is processed into information, which is used to guarantee evidence-based practice, which leads to decision support used for practice (Thede & Schwiran, 2015).

> "EHRs should be designed to provide practitioners with the ability to reflect accurately on their practice. Instead of relying on memory, which may often be selective, the ability to view data in the aggregate about patients for whom nurses provided care would allow nurses to be truly reflective of their practice. This ability could also create more interest among nurses in participating in nursing research." (Thede & Schwiran, 2015)

Next, we will compare electronic medical records with electronic health records and electronic patient records; discuss the importance of the clinical nurse's role in the selection of a clinical information system process; discuss the concept of workflow analysis as it relates to nursing care; compare the systems life cycle with the nursing process; discuss the role of the super-user in the systems life cycle; display adherence to HIPAA regulations when working with health information; discuss how a business continuity plan mitigates risk, and share a Web address—an additional learning resource for nursing students.

ELECTRONIC MEDICAL RECORDS (EMR)

Electronic medical records (EMR) are the digital accumulation of information generated during patients' encounter with health systems, whether it be immunization in the clinic or admission to the hospital emergency room for an appendectomy, or a visit to the doctor's office for a colonoscopy. It replaces the old way of keeping patients' records in papers and charts. Prior to this time, patients could have up to four manila folders in their medical record, depending on number of admissions and clinic visits. The information generated could not be shared with other outside health agencies. Now, with EMR, all the visits and encounters for different health issues can be researched. In case of emergencies or disasters such as hurricane, flood, fire, and terrorism, where paper medical records were destroyed, it is difficult to know victims' medical history or medication. So, treating patients without past medical history may further jeopardize their overall health. But EMR will instantly show victims' medical histories.

Furthermore, with the data generated from EMR, providers could note or monitor patient's progress and retrogress over time, which could reveal which group of patients are due for screenings or lab tests and evaluations. However, EMR deals only with the medical aspect of the patient and does not leave the facility. Even in cases of consults to outside specialists, EMR information would have to be printed. That is, EMR is confined in the organization. EMR is mainly used by clinicians for diagnosing and treatment (Garrett & Seidman, 2011).

EMR uses special coding and vocabulary to note information of order entry and provide computerized order entry about the medication and pharmacy issues and other documentations. The computerized provider order entry is a system derived from the traditional way of the provider writing the order and a unit secretary or unit clerk transcribing the order. The difference here is that the provider enters the order directly to avoid errors such as wrong medication transcription and illegible hand writing, and for other disciplines such as nursing and pharmacy, noting the order directly as it was written. Providers-physicians, nurse practitioners, and physician assistants who have the privilege of writing orders are required to pay special attention to alerts such as medication incompatibility. This is another way EMR strives to eliminate errors, thereby preserving patient safety. If any provider chooses to override the alert, he or she is required to write an explanation for the override.

ELECTRONIC HEALTH RECORDS (EHR)

In an attempt to improve healthcare and patient safety, the innovative electronic health record (EHR) was created. EHR was first initiated by President George W. Bush in 2004 who also appointed the National Coordinator for Health Information Technology (NCHIT) to conduct a strategic plan (Sewell & Thede, 2013). Based on this plan and to greater extent the report and recommendations of the Institute of Medicine (IOM), EHR came about. EHR, a subset of electronic medical records (EMR), is a collaborative way to share information among healthcare workers, interdisciplinary teams, and patients and/or their families.

Prior to this era, other disciplines kept their own health records. Patients' medical records were kept in papers housed in folders and charts. In cases where papers were lost or damaged, during disaster and emergency, the documents could not be retrieved. There was also redundancy of information, writing same information over and over and the subsequent mistakes of patients' poor memory, making them unable to accurately recall past medical history, and of medication error stemming from misinterpretation due to poor hand writing. In addition, lack of understanding certain unpopular acronyms, for example morphine sulfate (MSO4) interpreted as magnesium sulfate (MSO4), giving the wrong dose of medication or giving medication to the wrong patient, and time lag from the point of diagnosis to implementation all are mitigated by EHR.

The benefit of EHR is so great and convincing that the federal government set up a large financial incentive through the Commissions for Medicaid and Medicare Services (CMS) for providers and healthcare agencies that meet the criteria for "meaningful use" (Saba & McCormick, 2011). "Meaningful use" refers to a set of goals to be achieved by using certified EHR to improve patient outcome. There is a quest to adopt EHR, to meet the dead line set by American Recovery and Reinvestment Act (ARRA) through the Health Information Technology for Economic and Clinical Health (HITECH) Act. The new era of healthcare information technology as enhanced by evidence-based practice and boosted by the Patient Protection and Affordability Care Act (PPACA) is here to stay, but the end users', nurses, workflow and their monumental input to overall patient favorable outcome were not fully represented. There is a need to include all team care in the redesign and implementation of workflow process from start to finish for best patient outcome. In the same token, nurses need to step up in acquiring the knowledge needed to lead in the healthcare information-driven market place.

Electronic health records (EHR), a subset of EMR, on the other hand, are transportable collections of patients' health information that is shared among other healthcare agencies that initially collected the information. EHR looks at the holistic aspect of the individual and not just the medical information as with the EMR. Thus, a provider in a nursing home, outpatient clinic, or hospital is able to see patients' overall health history. In other words, a patient's primary, secondary, and tertiary health information follows the patient wherever he or she goes. In a nutshell, sharing of information across all providers taking care of the individual within and outside an organization, and even outside state interoperability, is what sets EHR apart from EMR.

Furthermore, EHR utilizes clinical data architecture (CDA). CDA is formulated by the health level 7 (HL7) a common clinical set of documents used to show simple standards for clinical documents. It has three levels and uses coding. For example, the patient's first name could have a code tagged to the name that the machine can read. The tag could represent items such as demography, medication, vital signs, etc., and only designated healthcare workers could understand what it means. The CDA shows how information should be shared. Another document type used with EHR is the continuity of care document (CCD). CCD uses a CDA specific set up to vividly provide patient health information relating to insurance coverage, diagnosis, medication, and allergies. While CDA provides how information is shared, CCD provides what information to be shared with EHRs.

Both EMRs and EHRs help providers have real-time accurate information of patients. For example, a provider can note the result of the lab it ordered for a patient last week because the lab attendant enters the result in the repository as soon as the lab was ran. EHRs will enhance safer treatment of patients during emergency or disaster because they take just a click of the button to see patients' health records. Pharmacies will readily see all patients' medication and will be able to note adverse effects and contraindication of medications. EHRs will make it easier to note trends and or outbreaks and use trends to effect change. EHRs complement evidence-based practice, and electronic health information exchange (HIE) is an important tool enabling quality care delivery in the communities across the country. According to the Office of the National Coordinator for Health Information Technology (2013):

> HIE is defined as the secure electronic movement of health-related information among health care entities according to nationally recognized standards. Traditionally, patient health information has been difficult to share. It is

done using manual and often time-consuming processes that require active coordination between the patient and provider teams and may involve the completion of numerous forms with mail and fax-based exchange of hard-copy health information. Electronic HIE allows patient health information to be shared across health care providers and institutions securely and efficiently, regardless of geographic or organizational boundaries. It allows information to follow patients across health care settings and visits. Prepared with timely, comprehensive, and up-to-date information on which to base care decisions, providers can improve both direct care delivery and the coordination of care across care settings. (ONCHIT, 2013, p. 1)

Another advantage of information sharing is that it makes departments proactive. When the information required for a patient's treatment is available at the right time, the treatment is effectively and timely managed with proven success. This is an opportunity of which most healthcare organizations avail themselves by looping and pairing the information in the sectional order. Another corollary advantage, according to Deborah Zarin (the director at the National Library of Medicine), is that information sharing brings transparency in healthcare operations (National Academy of Sciences, 2013). It brings transparency to how well patients are provided care and treatment. Information sharing also gives the opportunity for patients' retrospective analyses, as it allows the data exchange of patients' past records and trials. Although there are great opportunities in the availability and ability to share electronic health information, its effectiveness depends on the organization's competency to organize and utilize these great opportunities (National Academy of Sciences, 2013).

In the contemporary trend, if an organization is trusted, it is accredited by its patients and by its people. It is immensely important that these organizations work hard to maintain the trust of patients by transmitting their information safely and securely (Croskerry & Cosby, 2009). In recent practice, it has been found that healthcare centers keep patients' information accessible. They keep the information open to the departmental level to make patient's care efficient. It is the requirement of healthcare networks that they have quick and easy access to patient's private information. This may include patients' personal records of medications and records of treatment and disease. To make sure that the internal operations of healthcare are effective, accessible information is an important feature of healthcare electronic system. This is what improves the quality of service in healthcare and the efficiency of electronic networks that gives push to the entire healthcare operation (Croskerry & Cosby, 2009). From modern practices in healthcare, it can be assessed that organizations are centered on the quality of care. To get higher quality, organizations utilize their electronic healthcare system, which transmits the information purposively and with high protection (American Medical Association, 2013).

Having discussed the risks and the opportunities of clinical data sharing within healthcare systems and organizations and how they affect the privacy and confidentiality of patients, this paper will now discuss how interoperability affects the sharing of patient healthcare information.

In healthcare, information is mostly shared by means of paired sub-grouped systems. Such systems are heterogeneous and are of dissimilar nature. To loop such systems to one central objective (information sharing) is a challenge for healthcare organizations and could lead to major volume of patients at a single time of operation. Such systems are unlike in their content, information, and output and multiple looping is required to pass on the information efficiently. In fact, it is the ability of an electronic health information system that incorporates all the heterogeneous subsystems at one time. Getting aligning to subsystems is a major challenge for the main system, as it requires the diversity and flexibility of the system to get adjusted with the other subsystems (Tan & Payton, 2012).

To improve in health management and in the preventive care section, organizations have to deal with the interoperable environment, which is based on association of departments, hospitals, and their close electronic networks (Tan & Payton, 2012). The challenge, here, for healthcare organizations is of interaction and communication as each unit (system) is working independently from the other unit or system. For example, in hospitals there are wards of oncology, cardio, orthopedics, and surgical units, to mention but a few, where each ward/unit is carrying independent information with respect to the other ward/unit that is carrying dissimilar information. Communicating such dissimilar information is a challenge as it requires the flexibility of the system to get the information transferred. Without communicating information, it is difficult to improve the overall efficiency of the organization and the preventive care of the health management sections (Tan & Payton, 2012). The discussion in the next paragraph will be on workflow and redesigned and clinical documentation systems.

Healthcare workflow redesign refers to the alteration of the information flow pattern. The pattern of the information, if changed, in healthcare means that the process flow has been redesigned or restructured. This changing pattern of information and process is what demonstrates the modification of the workflow infrastructure in healthcare. It is the amendment in the documentation system that results through healthcare workflow redesign. The objective in the redesign is to improve the process of information flow (Chaiken, 2011). If flow of information is not interrupted, it can increase the overall pace of a healthcare organization. Redesigning means that the direction of flow of information has been changed, with an objective to make information more purposive and objective. In healthcare, departments are interlinked and work in a synchronized manner, which requires the information to flow in the right direction. Synchronization of data is only possible if the layout of the information system is redesigned or restructured (Chaiken, 2011).

The example of National Health Authority can be taken in this respect—an organization that transformed the entire IT setup. Keeping innovation and advancement as key objectives, the leadership at National Health Services (NHS) transformed its documentation system. The organization modified its workflows by converting all the clinical manual operations into automated ones (Triggle, 2013). From transcription procedures to patient care record procedures, all are automated in the NHS. Being one of the largest public healthcare organizations, NHS modified its modes of operation. The organization was modified with the administration documentation processes and clinical information patterns, giving room to the organization's individuals to perform and to lead. Efficiency became the motive of the organization when its IT system was transformed and modified (Triggle, 2013).

It is through workflow redesign that NHS is able to bring quality care for patients coming up in large numbers. All the enrolled regional patients who are carrying health insurance or financial insurance are brought for treatment in NHS. The organization upholds a larger set of data, allowing patients to get the treatment quickly, adequately, and in a smooth manner. Administrative delays and delays in the process flow are being avoided because NHS has been quite successful in adapting change in its documentation system. The documentation system is aligned to all the subsystems of the organization, which has made the organization fast, collaborative, and informative. All these make NHS the best example for the effectiveness of workflow redesign and how it operates. Having achieved this milestone of successfully redesigning a workflow that makes it easy to access patients' information from one unit or hospital to another, what are the necessary steps that must be taken by the organization to ensure that patients' safety is maintained while using healthcare information technology?

EHR AND PATIENT SAFETY

In contemporary healthcare practice, organizations are more concerned about "patients' safety." To achieve this goal, organizations have an electronic healthcare information system, which is a troubleshooter of almost all the major problems of a healthcare organization. To address the core objective of patient safety, organizations entail two more objectives: building a flexible decision support system and minimizing medical errors (Croskerry & Cosby, 2009). After the two primary goals are achieved by monitoring compliance, minimizing documentation lags, and coordinating care among departments, the patient safety objective is quite inevitably achieved. The EMR (electronic medical record) systems make this objective achievable. The systems ensure staff convenience and patient convenience by providing service providers quick access to information. Departmental delays, which are root causes to patients' accidents and inconvenience, are successfully avoided through EMRs. Such systems are highly coordinative and solve problems and risks of patients (Savage & Ford, 2008).

This content has argued extensively on the importance of electronic data sharing, the significance of protecting patients' privacy and confidentiality, and how the database is built, structured, and redesigned to provide quality care and safety for patients. However, not much has been said on how to protect these devices that store patients' information. Therefore, what follows will discuss the security measures that the healthcare institutions and system need to take to ensure that their electronic devices that store patients' information are not hijacked by unauthorized users or professional hijackers.

EHR SECURITY MEASURES

In healthcare organizations, securing patients' information is the most important task. If a hospital or a healthcare center is not able to secure its patients' personal information, it can get discredited by the government or the patients who are part of the organization's system (Shoniregun & Dube, 2010). For this reason, administrators and managers in healthcare emphasize the need to secure their healthcare networks. One method of securing network devices is by keeping a strong password. Passwords are used to secure confidential information of the organization and the information that is not in regular use. Main servers of the healthcare network can be secured through a strong password (Shoniregun & Dube, 2010). There are two strong passwords recommended for healthcare network security: namely XKCD passwords and Diceware encrypting.

The XKCD password is a proposition brought by Randall Munroe (roboticist and programmer at NASA). The password is based on four randomly selected common words. It is a strong password for protecting healthcare servers as it strongly restricts the brute forces. The password is easy to memorize as it is formulized on the basis of common words and with strong combinations to increase bits of entropy (Shoniregun & Dube, 2010). The higher the number of entropy, the more time a brute requires for breaking the password. Four randomly selected words keep a minimum of 44 combinations that, if get powered up with two, will make the password highly protected. The XKCD password is highly recommended for protecting main servers in healthcare, which are not in open use and keep patients' information confidential (Shoniregun & Dube, 2010).

Diceware encrypting is another strong password based on numeric organization. A dice is used in diceware encrypting. Rolling the dice five times assembles a strong five-digit password (Shoniregun & Dube, 2010). The combination does not end there, as the digit numbers are checked on the English coded list. The list translates the numbers to letters and produces an effective and highly protective password. The password is recommended for protecting healthcare mainframes. Safeguarding patients' personal information can be made possible through encrypted diceware. Network administrators can also apply the encrypted combination, giving basic protection to their desktop computers (Cheswick, 2003).

Healthcare administrators should also keep antivirus software for protecting the servers from virus intrusion (Shoniregun & Dube, 2010). A regular check should be made on protected computers, and servers should be updated with combinations of passwords. This enhances the security and protection of healthcare servers and networks (Shoniregun & Dube, 2010).

This section has showcased the challenges and risks that are embedded in the use of electronic data storing and sharing. It pointed out some of the risks such as patient identity exposure, identity mismatch or conflict, and data stealing and violation of patient privacy and confidentiality and the simultaneous risks of identity fraud, distortion of patients' healthcare records, and distortion of patients' medication records.

IT managers in healthcare organizations face these challenges while employing the benefits of being able to share patient data electronically and offer some recommendations on how to mitigate the effect of these challenges. If the healthcare systems and institutions' databases are protected with formidable passwords and workflow is redesigned to meet their needs, their staff would electronically share and use patient clinical data in such a way that it would not only enhance their effectiveness in caring for patients, but their ability to protect the privacy and confidentiality of their patients would be equal to none. In fact, their databases would be safe havens for the preservation and protection of patients' clinical information and their hospitals would be recognized as first in saving patients' lives.

NURSING AND EHR

When electronic health records (EHR) were first developed and implemented, healthcare professionals had no idea how this tool would affect the world. These advantages are used today to promote health and prevent illness as the population continues to grow exponentially. EHRs have many general benefits, as well specific benefits for nurses, healthcare providers, the healthcare enterprise, and payers (Hebda & Czar, 2009). With these benefits, we can detect problems in advance and intervene appropriately.

The electronic health record has benefits for providers and patients. First, it gives providers easy access to information needed to diagnose and improve outcomes for patients in emergency and nonemergency situations. Subsequently, it allows information to be easily shared among hospitals and other healthcare facilities. Improved communication gives rise to safer and better care. In addition, the use of an EHR can save space and time and preserve the environment by reducing the amount of paper used for storage. The utilization of EHR allows healthcare providers to write orders for patients, all while storing those orders without using much physical space. Furthermore, before the patient reaches the pharmacy, the pharmacy can receive a doctor's order and have it ready, saving time. The EHR helps protect patients' medical information with the use of a protected password. Information in the EHR can be retrieved in some situations such as destruction or fire because the information can easily be backed up and saved on alternate systems. In addition, the EHR could be used to enhance the environmentally sound healthcare sector if they could be expanded to change workflows and care delivery, rather than just a substitute for paper records" (Finney et al., 2011).

Although electronic health records have several generalized benefits associated with the healthcare industry, there are also specific nursing benefits that EHRs bring. EHRs help to make the job of nursing just that much easier in several different ways. EHRs help with the collection and storage of data. When using EHRs, a patient's current data, along with data from previous events, are stored in the EHR. With both sets of data being in the same database, it makes it easier for nurses to go back and compare data (Hebda & Czar, 2009). EHRs also allow nurses to have a continuous record of a client's education and their learning responses (Hebda & Czar, 2009). Another benefit of EHRs is the elimination of data repetition such as in baseline demographic data. EHRs also help nurses in more ways than just specific client care. All data recorded in the EHRs can be accessed by anyone with access to the EHR system, allowing for the improvement of quality of data research and data access (Hebda & Czar, 2009). The improvement of documentation, quality of care, and automatic use of critical and clinical pathways are another extraordinary nursing benefit that EHRs bring to the table (Hebda & Czar, 2009). As EHRs have already benefited the nursing profession with so much already, they can also help with research derived through the database and can give information that makes the jobs of administrators and clinicians easier (Hebda & Czar, 2009). The most useful element of EHRs for nurses is their ability to possess comprehensive information about the consumer in one centralized server and in handwriting translation (Orlovsky, 2011).

Maintaining electronic health records is beneficial to healthcare providers. Healthcare providers are interdisciplinary members and play a vital role in the treatment and diagnosis of disease. Imagine record keeping completely on traditional paper rather than electronic. In that case, the healthcare provider might be spending a lot of time and effort waiting for the old records to be delivered from the records department and accessing previous records or charting and documenting patient's conditions. Some key information might be lost from one visit to the next visit, thus placing the patient at a higher risk for a wrong diagnosis. It is less costly and improves the efficiency of billing. Better documenting and recording of diagnostic and treatment procedures, as well as that of the client's progress, enhances reimbursement for the hospital (Health It, 2012). Moreover, the EHR has more dynamic properties such as medical vocabulary, trends, clinical graphics, reporting tools on demand, and early warning systems if there are changes in patients' status. All these tools help to increase healthcare providers' performance.

Not only does the EHR benefit healthcare providers, but it also benefits the healthcare enterprise. Hebda and Czar (2009) list some of the benefits as in improved client record safety, enhanced communication, and efficient record management (Hebda & Czar, 2009). Protecting patients' privacy and securing their health information, including information in electronic health records, is a main piece to build trust that can show the potential benefits of electronic health information exchange.

> If individuals and other participants in a network lack trust in electronic exchange of information due to perceived or actual risks to electronic health information or the accuracy and completeness of such information, it may affect their willingness to disclose necessary health information and could have life-threatening consequences. (Health It, n.d.)

That also ties into effective communication; when a provider adds patient notes or lab test results to patient her, that information can be available to all healthcare providers authorized to view that particular patient record, so they can have access to the most up-to-date information about the patient's health in different health facilities. "Some healthcare providers may allow the patient to access their own health information directly, meaning no longer have to wait to hear back from care provider for information such as test results that are normal and may not require an explanation" (Health IT, n.d.). After all, this can also help to reduce paper work. By having electronic health records, patients do not have to answer the same questions about personal information and medical history multiple times or provide copies of their records every time they go to doctor visit or referral.

Faced with the numerous benefits provided by EHRs, most healthcare facilities should strive to acquire such systems and use them to support healthcare practice. However, Hebda and Czar (2009) warn us of the potential perils associated with "hasty decisions" about which specific system should be purchased, and how that system would then be integrated into daily care routines. Essentially, bad integration of an EHR system into any health practice may not provide all the benefits normally associated with it. Silow-Carroll,

Edwards, and Rodin (2012) enumerate some of the factors needing consideration before purchase of an EHR, including "vendor provision of technical support before, during, and after implementation" and "availability of upgrades that help hospitals meet meaningful-use guidelines" (Health IT, n.d.). An EHR system that is well maintained and flexible can provide the greatest benefits as it can be tailored to different tasks as the need arises. With that in mind, enough time should be allotted for planning and choosing an appropriate commercial electronic medical record if all benefits are to be removed.

The EHR is just another example of how computers and technology are helping people today. It is beneficial to everyone one in the healthcare system and allows information and data to be transcribed more easily, as well as accessed more effortlessly. It can help reduce errors throughout the system and makes processes speedier, which can help patients when there is an emergency. Instead of having to look through paper records in a chart that can be out of order or disorganized, the EHR can help quicken the process of finding the exact information that is needed. As knowledge, equipment, and technology grows, the future is looking brighter and more helpful to all involved with the new systems. It is all about bettering humanity and enhancing ways to speed up processes that will help improve human life and safety and give a better chance for a more healthy life.

Nurses are the largest provider of healthcare; in addition, they are the end users of EHR. Therefore, nurses should be at the forefront of selecting clinical information processes. The contribution of nurses to achieve the goals of patient safety and improved overall health outcome is unparalleled. Obviously, without nurses there would be no hospital, and the payment for nursing services accounts for the largest hospital expenditure. Again, nursing pioneers have helped to achieve the benefits of EHR since 2007 (Saba & McCormick, 2011). Nursing has professional information technologists whose potential is untapped. Besides, inpatient workflow is embedded in the nursing process, so nursing professionals (of course with IT experience) appointed to clinical system processes would richly enhance these projects. The nurse should enroll in nursing informatics programs and educational events. He or she should network and attend informatics outreach educational activities, ask questions, and listen to experts within the profession. The nurse also would be prepared to lead and become a change agent.

Lippincott's DocuCare was founded as faculty collaboration at the University of Tennessee, Knoxville. The Lippincott's DocuCare group was initially named iCare (Lippincott & Wilkins, 2012). The primary objective of this group was to develop educational health record for students' practice. The qualities of the electronic health records developed by iCare included affordability, the ability to prepare students for practice, and the ability to meet educational needs of the students. The need to enhance the educational EHR to fit the requirements of all programs led to collaboration between Lippincott Williams and Wilkins, with an objective of meeting documentation needs for preparing students for practice (Schwirian, 2013). The collaboration led to establishment of Lippincott's DocuCare team. The team is currently devoted to quality services and achieving the original goals of iCare. Lippincott's DocuCare has boosted the development of electronic health records for educational purposes (Lippincott & Wilkins, 2012). The success of Lippincott's DocuCare comes from the team's dedication to collect and store more than

150 patient records. These records contain a wide range of diseases and conditions across the lifespan and curriculum.

In 2013, an electronic health record tool for nursing students was developed by Elsevier Evolve for clinical, simulation and case scenarios. The tool gives students the foundation they need to be successful in today's modern and paperless healthcare environment. Simchart can also be integrated throughout the entire nursing program, from fundamentals through leadership. Simchart is an EHR tool specifically built as a teaching tool for nursing students in classrooms, simulation labs, and clinicals. In addition, it is loaded with pre-built unfolding case studies and integrated with clinical decision support tools (Elsevier-SimChart, 2017).

Cain and Haque (2008) define workflow as a map of an action plan or process designed to accomplish a task in less time that ultimately leads to consistency, safety, and reliability according to standard of practice. The nursing workflow is centralized in the nursing process: assessment, diagnosis, implementation, and evaluation. The nurses perform these activities to effect change in patient response. According to research, information cannot become knowledge by itself except with critical thinking and the cognitive, intellectual, and analytical ability of the nurse that transforms data collected into useful knowledge in EHR. The researcher emphasizes that processing information for delivering patient care should not deviate from workflow for best quality healthcare outcome (Whittenburg, 2010).

Again, nursing workflow is patient centric and therefore must be supported by EHR. The work flow could be accomplished by people or by electronics. For example, a computer on wheel (COW), which the nurse takes to patients' rooms to accomplish the processes of nursing practice, from assessment, that is weight and height, vital signs, intake and output etc., to evaluation, noting patient's response to pain medication or noting improvement in patient's temperature. The nurse being able to enter the information in EHR via COW while in the patient's room without interruption or returning to the nursing station to enter the data shows that COW is nursing workflow technology.

However, with **computerized physician order entry (CPOE),** nurses have to return to the nursing station with the vital signs, intake and output data, etc., and wait for their turn before entering the information in EHR terminal. In this case, electronic workflow is not completely enhanced by CPOE EHR application. Furthermore, nurses are at the forefront for the successful implementation of CPOE, due in large part to nurses holding the position to coordinate and communicate care. Therefore, understanding nurses' workflow in addition to order entry is quite essential.

System life cycle (SLC), which connotes a set of action from start to finish of a project, is congruent to nursing processes in that nursing processes begin with assessment and end with evaluation. But, before reaching evaluation, there may be a turn of events (for example, the patient may code), and even after reaching evaluation, if the outcome is unfavorable, the process is repeated with a different strategy that may yield a better outcome. For example, when a patient arrives in the hospital, a nurse assesses the patient including vital signs, BP (245/130) (assessment), etc. The patient is diagnosed with hypertensive crisis (diagnosis). The nurse initiates an antihypertensive drip according to order and protocol (implementation). BP may start dropping or fluctuating. However, if that medication does not work (bring the BP down) for the patient after a while (evaluation), the nurse and the physician may decide on another medication. Whichever antihypertensive that helped to normalize the patient's BP, the patient would be maintained on it.

In the same way, initializing system life cycles and planning project goals and scope needs and budget, as well as task, cost, and system specifics, signifies patient arrival to the hospital with a problem; then the patient is registered and insurance and payment options noted. The patient is triaged to see which department to send the patient and how urgent his or her condition is. The identified goal is to bring the BP back to normal. The patient is transferred to the critical care unit/coronary care unit (CCU) and the there is an initiation of the antihypertensive intravenous drip. Controlling the situation represents the frequent assessment of patient and monitoring of BP to note the therapeutic effect of the medication. Then, costs are finalized and the project is evaluated to measure the effectiveness of the medication and the patient outcome. If BP was normalized, the patient would be discharged; if not, the cycle resumes with a different strategy. Maintenance and continuous evaluation of the patient is an ongoing process. In all, the facility needs a strategic plan to streamline the actions needed to implement information systems.

Super-users are clinical nurses recruited from each unit where the system is implanted. Super-users have the capability to market the product and assist other end users with training, service, and implementation. They are the backbone to answer questions and to help others learn to use the system. Super-users are the change agents and are invaluable. They assist the rest of the staff to learn and implement the system process. The knowledge of HIPAA could not be over emphasized. Healthcare staff should endeavor to remember the security aspect of HIPAA. They should learn and use security features and strategies embedded in most handheld devices to prevent access to information such as encryption and passwords. Just as any other group of business entities have plan for emergencies, HIS management teams have plans to mitigate risks including backup plants for power outages with remote databases where all essential copies of the same software applications used in facilities are kept, including how to use them. Last, Lippincott Williams, and Wilkins established a website called "The Point" that has very useful health information ranging from books, EHR and other databases, and anatomy and physiology cards for both students and faculty.

E-PERSONAL HEALTH RECORDS

Aside from EMR and EHR is the electronic personal health record (ePHR). It is a person's own medical record as written and kept by the person. Due to memory failure or emergency situations, a patient may not be able to recall or accurately remember past medical history. That is, if the patient did not write down his or her medical history, even for a healthy individual, it is sometimes difficult to remember exact dates and times of health events. The person's individual record will not be of any good to the individual until the record is shared with the personal care provider (PCP).

The ePHR assists patients in maintaining their health record. It helps individuals take an active role in their healthcare decisions. Both provider and the patient can look at the record together, ask questions, clarify issues, and set and achieve goals. To fully engage consumers in ePHR, there has been recommendations to start consumer informatics and educate people from grade school.

Among the barriers to ePHR are (a) the difficulty for some providers to release autonomy, as they want to retain the old way of keeping the information; (b) the fear of releasing such information to a lay person, as with divulging information about psychiatrics to an individual who may not have any inclination of the disease process; and (c) fear of litigation.

EHR CHALLENGES

There is tremendous potential that the digitization of healthcare documentation promises to the healthcare industry. The problematic aspect of electronic healthcare records is the possibility of such records becoming a pervasive and powerful means of committing healthcare fraud. Healthcare providers sometimes use this advanced technology to interfere with the medical system, with the objective of obtaining payments to which they are not entitled. This becomes a possibility because the electronic health record can automatically generate deceptive patient histories. Doctors can also copy and paste the same results from examination for multiple clients. Investigation reports reveal that medical professionals hike their billings to the Medicare program by using remunerative billing codes through creating detailed patient files (Azari, Janeja, & Mohseni, 2012).

The use of electronic health records has led to increased number of hackers interested in patients' medical records. Hackers steal backup tapes that contain health insurance records for patients. The hackers are interested in finding the medical history and examinations of prominent people and military officials. The United States Department of Defense, for example, reported that a number of backup tapes were stolen from a contractor for TRICARE, an agency that provides health insurance to members of the armed forces (Azari, Janeja, & Mohseni, 2012). According to the reports, personal data and medical documents of 5 million patients who were treated in the military for 20 years was compromised during this incident.

LEGAL AND ETHICAL ISSUES OF USING TECHNOLOGY IN NURSING

Cambridge's *Dictionary of Philosophy* states that "ethics means the moral principles of a particular tradition, group or individual." In general, ethics is the rational, optimal, and appropriate decision brought on by the basis of common sense. However, this does not exclude the possibility of mistakes or destruction of ethics due to malicious intent. Ethics can be used in three related ways: philosophical ethics, religious ethics, and a moral code. Legal and ethical issues in nursing informatics involve many pressing issues such as the right of the consumer to choose or refuse treatment or the right to limit the level of suffering one will endure during any given healthcare treatment. The fast pace of healthcare technology and informatics has allowed for prolonged continuation of life. With many people living longer, the meaning of what is an acceptable quality of life continues to change. Technology and informatics continue to make healthcare delivery systems very challenging and complicated. For this reason, healthcare ethics, including nursing ethics, is no longer limited to philosophical issues. Rather, it is comprised of cost effectiveness and economic, medical, nursing, legal, and political issues. Nursing and medical ethics share many principles such as beneficence, non-malfeasance, and autonomy of the patient in care. However, nursing ethics emphasizes human dignity, collaborative care, and nurse-patient interpersonal relationships. Recently nursing ethics is shifting toward nurses' obligation to patients' rights. This is reflected in many professional nursing codes and ethics, including the code from the International Council of Nurses (Norris, 2002). To fully understand the critical issues of legal and ethics in nursing informatics, the critical content areas will be further explored as in nursing codes, ethics and informatics codes, privacy information breaches, HIPAA, telehealth issues with practice, implantable identification concerns, Web 2.0 applications' usage, and copyright issues.

There are similarities and differences between professional nursing codes of ethics and professional informatics associations' codes; the health informatics professionals play unique roles in the planning and delivery of healthcare services that are distinct from the roles of other professional informatics personnel working in different settings. One aspect of this uniqueness is the relationship and responsibilities between the electronic health record (EHR) and the patient. The electronic health record (EHR) provides information about patients and must be guarded, protected, and kept confidential, but, more importantly, it remains a vital basis for healthcare decisions that have a profound impact on the course of care for each patient. This unique position of the health informatics professional must balance ethical justification during care. The electronic health record (EHR) also provides raw data for decision making by the government, other agencies, and the healthcare institutions that provide care. The health informatics professional (HIP) and electronic health records (EHR) make it possible for the delivery of healthcare services to patients by facilitating the construction, maintenance, storage, access, use, and manipulation of electronic health records (EHR). Rules of ethical conduct for HIPs consists of six general rubrics, as follows:

- Subject-centered duties
- Duties for HCPs
- Duties for institutions/employers
- Duties for society
- Self-regarding duties
- Duties for the profession

National nursing associations have similar nursing codes of ethics, which are very similar in wording. All nurses must live by these rules that are set by their respective association and the International Council of Nurses. The nursing codes are open to interpretation. Violation of the codes can result in loss of practice privileges or suspension of licenses. Some of the codes utilized in health informatics relating to electronic health records are implied in the nursing codes; however, the nursing codes need to be clear because of the ever-changing informatics technology. Nurses, healthcare practitioners, and health informatics practitioners have the same responsibility of guarding consumers' privacy, autonomy, confidentiality, and rights. According to the American Nurses Association Code of Ethics, provisions 3, 5, 7 and 8, nurses also have the professional responsibility to be competent through continued education and by contributing to professional scholarships and providing correct health information to the consumers and the public. These provisions are also important for health informatics professionals to protect healthcare consumers and the public at large.

Breaches of private information can occur by the following:

- Loss or theft of electronic devices and/or gargets such as laptops and flash drives or backup devices, especially with unencrypted data
- Computer viruses
- Hackers
- Systems break down (e.g., the computer electrical system broke down at the Transport Safety Administration (TSA), recently and all data was lost)

Strengths and Weaknesses of the Health Insurance Portability and Accountability Act (HIPAA) of 1996

The Health Insurance Portability and Accountability Act (HIPAA) of 1996 (Public Law 104–191) was enacted to ensure the protection, privacy, confidentiality, and security of patients' health information. All forms of documentation methods are covered under this law (i.e., verbal, electronic, and/or paper formats). The law remains applicable to all electronically transmitted and maintained healthcare information. HIPAA standards also include accessibility restriction to individually identifiable healthcare information, including disclosure and use of information. It also imposes administrative restrictions such as educational training, accreditation compliance, and enforcement of HIPAA laws. With the protection the law provides with regards to privacy of health information, it is not applicable to all domains that keep medical records, especially those domains that only keep medical records from healthcare providers outside of the domains. The law does not cover all private healthcare information. HIPAA only covers three categories of healthcare providers:

- Health plans
- Fee-for-service healthcare providers
- Healthcare clearing houses that bill CMS electronically for reimbursements of services

Telehealth Issues Associated with Practicing Nursing across State Lines

Telecommunication technologies have provided the avenue for telehealth, which allows two or more healthcare clinicians to care for a patient simultaneously by sharing pertinent information about the patient. It can also be very complicated such as performing robotic surgery virtually between two facilities or across the ocean. Telehealth technology gave a new paradigm to healthcare services. It has provided a way to get healthcare services to patients between different geographical locations and jurisdictions, especially in remote regions that lack healthcare clinicians and/or specialists for consumers. As a result of this technology and different modalities of delivering healthcare, quality of life has improved.

However, the question of interstate or intercontinental clinical practice and licensure became an obvious dilemma for many states in the United States and around the globe (Maheu, Whitten, & Allen, 2001).

One of the pressing questions to the dilemma is where the clinician should be licensed if the patient and healthcare provider are in different geographical locations at the time the care is rendered. The flip side of the question is whether the healthcare provider should be licensed in the state or geographical location of the patient, the consumer of healthcare. The American Telemedicine Association (ATA) and the American Medical Association (AMA) were the first healthcare professional associations to shed light on how to answer these questions ethically and professionally. Both organizations support the licensure to be handled at the state level in the United States.

In 1996, the Federation of State Medical Boards produced the conceptual frame work on which the restricted license was created, thereby allowing interstate telemedicine practices. The ultimate decision to adapt the restricted licensure policy was left at the discretion of each state. Two years later, in 1998, the National Council of State Boards of Nursing (NCSBN) endorsed the Nurse Licensure Compact (NLC) as a frame work for interstate nursing practices. The Nurse Licensure Compact (NLC) covers the registered nurse (RN), licensed practical nurse (LPN), and vocational nurse (VN) practices licensure. Under this interstate licensure agreement between the states, any of these categories of nurses, with valid license, can practice electronically and/or physically in all the states on the agreement compact. Based on the NLC mandate, personal licensure data must be coordinated with the compact states and stored electronically in a licensure information system (LIS).

In 2007, the American Telehealth Association (ATA) endorsed the collaborative effort agreement between states for implementation of interstate licensure for healthcare providers within the United States (Olmeda, 2000). In 2002, the National Council of Board of Nurses (NCBN) also adopted the same conceptual framework with the Nurse Licensure Compact for the advanced practice nurses (APRNs) for those states that have already implemented the Nurse Licensure Compact (NLC).

Pros and Cons of the Implantable Patient Identifier Using Radio Frequency Identification Microchip Technology

The technology that allows the use of electromagnetic fields to transfer pertinent data for the sole purpose of identification of an object or human that it is attached to is known as the radio-frequency identification (RFID). Currently, implantable patient identifiers using radio frequency identification microchip technology are being used in healthcare. Subdermal implant of radio-frequency identification (RFID) can be surgically implanted in the body. The RFID contains a unique identification number that can be linked to external databases for information on the person, such as personal identification, medical conditions, allergies, medical and family history, medications, etc. The RFID is wireless and can be used for automatically tracking tags and transferring data. The tags contain electronically stored information. Some tags are powered by electromagnetic induction via the electromagnetic fields. Other tags are powered by batteries or electromagnetic radiation (i.e., UHF radio waves). The reading can be achieved within very little range because the tag may be invisible to the reader as it is embedded in the tracked object, different from the bar code seen on the involved merchandise item. Automatic identification and data capture (AIDC) is a technological tool which provides direct data entry to a computer, or other micro-processor controlled system, without resorting to manual methods of data entry (Automatic identification and data capture) (AIDC, 2018). Today, data collection and maintenance is increasingly being automated to the point where AIDC systems can solely function without depending on human operators for basic data identification and capture.

Many industries are now using radio-frequency identification (RFID). Examples of these industries are automobile, pharmaceutical and livestock industries. Gas production industries also use the RFID tags on personnel for safety purposes, especially with the off-shore oil and gas platforms. These tags allow them to be located quickly all the time in the case of emergencies. Radio-frequency identification (RFID) is now being attached to clothing to track movement. This technology has improved the bottom line and safety for businesses by promoting efficiency and reducing theft and/or errors.

In the very near future, it is anticipated that GPS-enabled chip digital tools will enable remotely located individuals to be physically present by latitude, longitude, altitude, speed, and direction of movement (Wikipedia, 2018). If the GPS becomes implantable, it could allow the police and/or government to locate fugitives, criminals, child abusers, child abductors, and missing persons. These are good things; however, the technology will allow no place for innocent people to hide either. Anyone could then be located anywhere in the world.

The implantable devices are unencrypted; therefore, they are easily tampered with by being vulnerable to third-party readers. However, there are cons when it comes to implantation devices to human beings. These problems are as follows:

- Loss of privacy in healthcare data and medical records that may lead to cloning people and discrimination of people with catastrophic diseases such as cancer and HIV/AIDS
- Subcutaneous sarcomas (i.e., cancer)
- Electrical hazards
- Micro-resonance imaging (MRI) incompatibility
- Adverse tissue reaction
- Migration of the implanted transponder
- Societal and religious criticism, from Abrahamic religions through Christianity and Islam
- Prohibition by some states

Examples of Appropriate and Inappropriate Professional Nurse Use of Web 2.0 Applications

Web 2.0 is a technological application that not only allows users to retrieve information, but also provide the interface and software and storage facilities via the browser that allows for networking. One of the major features of Web 2.0 is social networking sites. This technology allows users to input information on media such as Facebook. Web 2.0

applications include blogs, videos, pictures, Facebook, Google, podcasts, and Yahoo. All these media are open to the world and the information posted is seen worldwide. It is therefore imperative for the nurse-user to be ethical in the process of posting anything.

In utilization of social media, the nurse must take into consideration his or her patients' confidentiality, privacy, and autonomy during and after caring for the patient. The nurse must also remember, at all times, that the policy and procedure of his or her work place as it relates to patient care and the utilization of social media. Quite a lot of people have encountered serious problems and/or experienced personal and professional losses based on what they have posted about themselves and/or others (Olmeda, 2000).

In using social media, nurses must not include any demographic information or data that will identify the person or patient. The nurse must also not include any identifying or negative information about his or her customers, peers, subordinates, employer, or any other work associates. Every post must be indicative of personal respect and respect for others, especially those whose care are entrusted to the healthcare practitioners, including nurses. Any posting must be done with utmost professionalism, moral standards, and code of ethics and follow the rules of the law.

Copyright Law Activities Associated with the Scholarship of Professional Publications by Nurses

The original creator of any work (e.g., books, articles, etc.) is given the exclusive rights of the intellectual property by copyright. The right is given for a limited length of time and gives credit for the work to the copyright holder. The original creator of the work will also have the right to determine who may adapt and/or perform the work and who may receive financial and/or other benefits from the said work. Copyright laws in the United Stated have been transformed to include fixed tangible media, even when not registered with the appropriate government agencies. The copyright registration allows for the original creator of any work under the copyright law to sue for unlawful or unfair utilization of his or her work. It is important for nurses to be aware of copyright laws. It will be deemed unethical and unprofessional for nurses to use the work of another person without respect for "intellectual property" laws, and plagiarism can now be detected by the use of computer software programs or search engines.

Legal and ethical issues in nursing informatics are complex and evolving at rapid rates and have been challenging; however, the healthcare organizations, including the regulating boards of the nursing profession, are still struggling to regulate their respective ethical codes. It will be necessary for these organizations to continue to update their respective codes of ethics and laws as the informatics technology continues to evolve at an alarming rate to constantly address the issues of patients' autonomy, confidentiality of data and health information, and invasion of privacy (McAfee, 2006). The use of unencrypted implantable devices is known to be easily tampered with because of the vulnerability of being stolen by a third party. The cons to using implantable devices in human beings are many, including but not limited to the loss of privacy in healthcare data and medical records, discrimination of people with catastrophic diseases such as cancer and HIV/AIDS, subcutaneous sarcomas (i.e., cancer, electrical hazards, especially with high voltage devices), micro-resonance imaging (MRI) incompatibility, adverse tissue reaction, migration of implanted transponders, and societal and religious criticism.

Each board of nurses is regulated by each state of the union. The differences in the regulation of nursing practices from state to state make it difficult to have a uniform statue to govern the interstate licensure of nurses. Only 24 states board have a collaborative agreement on Nurse Licensure Compact (NLC).

The legal and ethical issues are more important in nursing and all other healthcare professions because of the ever-evolving informatics and copyright laws. Nurses must play their part in staying abreast of the new laws and boundaries that the new field of informatics and electronic healthcare records are imposing on how healthcare delivery systems are managed (Simpson, 2006). The past of healthcare delivery systems was interesting, but the future is exciting. The focus of care is continuously challenged to be better, resulting in the shifting of ethics, from abstract principles to the unique demands of specific situations and interpersonal relationships between healthcare consumers and providers, including compassion, dignity, and empathy.

Information technology, including EMR, EHR, and ePHR, are among the revolutionary trends in healthcare arena. The overarching need for EHR is patient safety. The impact of EHR is a phenomenon; the federal government is rewarding healthcare agencies for utilizing it for improved patient outcome and later penalizing it for not being used. Advanced and higher education for nurses is more critical now than ever. With EHR, EBP, PPACA, information literacy, and technology, nurses should position themselves to lead the revolution. Nurses are pioneers in the progress made with quality patient outcome. They are the architect in implementing CPOE because they are responsible for communicating data that becomes information, knowledge, and then wisdom. Nursing workflow based on nursing processes that are guided by nursing practice accomplishes patients' goals, which are consistency, reliability, and safety. There is need for process redesign, which would include all members of the healthcare team for effective interoperability.

Because nurses are the largest set of healthcare providers and most EHR users, and the fact that interoperable workflow design mimics nursing processes and system life cycles, nurses should be represented and consulted with regarding system processing and redesign. Nurses also should step up in the information technology arena to be competent and versatile with the use of computer information technology. It is a new world of information technology. The game changer is informatics; nurses should not be left out in the information technology-driven healthcare market place.

Health Information Security Concepts Continues

HIPAA

Why is the use of information practices in healthcare institutions important? Well, you cannot have confidentiality without information security. An act of balance should always be present with the ease of access to patient health information for prompt medical and maintenance of information security to maintain confidentiality of patient's' health information. Studies have ascertained that information security should be correlated to the risk and the value of values being protected (Kurtz, 2009). The need to secure and maintain confidentiality of patients' medical information has led to the institution of the Health Insurance Portability Accountability Act (HIPAA) in 1996. Even though HIPAA is widely used across the country, how it is demonstrated in each facility is uniquely individual. For example, one healthcare institution may practice patient confidentiality techniques differently compared to another institution. But all healthcare institutions must abide by the rules set in place by HIPAA. The correct implementation of the standard of confidentiality is determined and implemented by the administration and information security departments.

In our group case study, the nurse manager loads a copy of the spreadsheet program that she uses at home onto one of the unit's PCs. Although the institution has a well-publicized policy against the use of unauthorized and unlicensed software copies, the nurse manager continues to download the software despite the policies set in place by the institution. Regardless of what information is being inputted, the nurse manager's behavior is inappropriate. She is possibly jeopardizing hundreds of patients' files by making the institution's computers vulnerable to possible unauthorized outside access. The nurse manager may think she is being productive, but she is blatantly going against proper protocol. Throughout the remainder of this paper, we will elaborate on privacy, confidentiality and security related to patient health information as well as HIPAA, administrative roles, risk factors, and security management.

Before moving to the roles of HIPAA and administrative departments, we must first define and differentiate between privacy, confidentiality, and security. Though all three have similar characteristics, they possess many differentiating aspects. Privacy is having control over the exposure of self or personal information, as well as freedom from intrusion (Hebda & Czar, 2012). With that said, privacy is usually defined by the individual divulging the information. For example, the person disclosing the information has the right to determine what information is to be shared, how it is utilized, and how and what information is made available. Next, confidentiality is when a relationship has been established and where private information is exchanged (Hebda & Czar, 2012). For example, in the relationship between the nurse and patient, the nurse establishes trust with the patient. By establishing trust, the patient shares private information with the expectation that what has been said will be kept confidential from those who are not partaking in care. This is one reason why HIPAA was instituted. HIPAA is a constant reminder to healthcare professionals of the prohibition of disclosing information about a client's health status to other parties without proper consent. Lastly, information security is defined as the protection of information against threats to its integrity, accidental disclosure, or availability (Hebda & Czar, 2012). The security of information has been better protected through the use of automated records that can only be viewed by a person who is privileged and has an access code. By taking these steps, the nurse and other healthcare professionals are able to provide continued quality, safe, and holistic care.

HIPAA is an established public standard for the protection of individuals' personal health information (PHI). It addresses the usage and revelation of individuals' health information, as well as privacy rights, to understand and control how their health information is utilized. The main purpose of instituting the HIPAA Privacy Rule is to assure that individual health information is protected appropriately, while permitting circulation of health information needed to provide enhanced quality care and to protect the health and well-being of the public (U.S. Department of Health and Human Services, 2003). Protection of client privacy and confidentiality serves as one on the many keys to client treatment and it is the client's right. The client is entitled to the protection of his or her privacy, confidentiality, and continued maintenance of the integrity of their information. It is crucial that once a client discloses confidential information, it is shared only with those who require it for client treatment and care (U.S. Department of Health and Human Services, 2003).

In addition to privacy, confidentiality, and information security, it is just as important to be ethical when caring for patient information. Ethics is a set of rules that are put in place by administrators of the institution and should be followed by all personnel when carrying out services to patients to maintain a professional, safe, and secure healthcare environment. To maintain the security of patient information and employee communication, it is the responsibility of administration to have all security measures in place to prevent security breaches, which may include breaches of patient confidentiality. Ways to help prevent breaches in confidentiality are by implementing security measures, such as monitoring system activities of various users with different levels of access. It is the healthcare administrator's duty to formulate protocols and procedures to be followed by all staff members working in the facility. It is imperative that institutional leaders must ensure that security awareness training are in place for all the stakeholders, employees, students, consultants, and contractors, because privacy and security are responsibilities shared by everyone in the organization (Hebda & Czar, 2012). Maintaining confidentiality in an institution goes beyond patient care; it is a representation of the institution as a whole in a business aspect. The administration department also partners with information security to make sure client information is protected at all times. By partnering, they are able to enhance security of information. It is important for administration to be strong in policies and procedures to continually maintain the security of patient health information.

With the advances of technology, it is becoming somewhat easier to promote and maintain confidentiality in the healthcare setting. Ensuring the client's privacy is a key component. This is especially true when dealing with patient information and technological advances. As nurses, we are all advocates of the client and it is our duty to secure their information and protect their rights (Hanks, 2010). We must also act on behalf of our clients. The use of biometrics in the healthcare setting would improve client information security because biological identification traits such as voice, fingerprint, or even iris scan identification would need to be used, making it more difficult for unauthorized personnel to gain access to sensitive information (Hanks, 2010).

Finally, referencing back to the case study looked at earlier, if the institution has a well-publicized policy against the use of unauthorized, unlicensed software copies, there is no reason why this set standard should be violated. There are many laws put into place so that the patient's information is confidential, and privacy is the last thing a patient should have to worry about when entering a healthcare facility. It is the healthcare facilities, as well as the nurse's, duty to ensure the clients' safety and provide them with the most efficient quality care. By having a good foundational relationship with your client, you can help in more ways than one. Having a trusting relationship with your client can prove to be beneficial, especially when it comes to helping him or her return to a healthier state. As nurses, we are the patient's last resort, their number-one advocate, and we should always respect and uphold, and not take lightly, their rights in regards to privacy and confidentiality.

Case #2: Potential Problems of Electronic Healthcare Systems

In most of the under-developed world where the only means of keeping medical records and/or patients' medical history is through hand-written reports, continuity of all patients' care, but more especially the most critical and vulnerable ones, are at best compromised and at worst lead to death. A case that readily comes to mind was an incident that happened with the father of a friend of mine, Mr. P. This patient had chronic obstructive pulmonary disease and some allergy history, but when he was being transported from the hospital in his little city to another bigger hospital in an urban area, the hospital staff that did the transfer forgot to bring the patient's medical file with them. By the time they realized it, they had already reached the hospital. Although they swiftly sent someone to rush back to bring the patient's medical file, the physician at the emergency department, unaware of the patient's allergy gave patient medications that caused an allergic reaction. Consequently, it caused the patient anaphylaxis/cardiac arrest; the patient went into a coma and died.

Mr. P's life and the lives of many others in similar situations would have been saved if access to the sophisticated electronic information technology system that is prevalent in most Western and developed worlds was available. Electronic information technology has a proven record of assisting healthcare organizations to record, maintain, and manage patients' clinical data between different institutions and systems in a timely manner. On a similar note, the ability to effectively share patients' clinical data electronically is one of the most leading productive tools that has saved many lives, has led to patient satisfaction and trust, and has led to a higher rating of healthcare institutions and systems. It does this by providing enhanced, correct, and prompt communication to other medical staff and institutions that are involved in providing care to patients, especially in the most critical situations where the survival of patients depends on seconds.

However, these and other benefits of electronic clinical data sharing between different healthcare systems and institutions have not come without a cost. One of the leading shortcomings or disadvantages of the electronic clinical data sharing is the violation of patients' privacy and confidentiality. While it may be a legitimate argument to say that the benefits of saving patients' lives outweigh the damage or harm that the violation of privacy and confidentiality may cause (depending on who you asked), the rate at which this violation occurs could at worst be minimized and at best be eradicated from the list of medical malpractices if healthcare institutions manage and protect their database properly by using the tools and formidable passwords and passwords setting techniques that are available to them.

Advanced Electronic Health Records

As the trend of electronic health records continues to infiltrate all levels of healthcare (primary, secondary, and tertiary) the outlook of electronic health information systems has begun to shift focus to a more specialized approach. According to Hall, Poole, and Clayton (2013),

Healthcare leaders as well as clinicians need a more sophisticated business intelligence tools to improve decisions and performance. It is further articulated that healthcare leaders must focus on actively improving quality by doing better with less, partnering with other providers to meet the demands for innovation and personalized medicine while complying with increasing regulatory and enforcement activities. (p. 419–426)

This has increased the pressure on healthcare facilities to achieve better outcomes. The use of information systems improves providers' ability to make informed timely decisions (Abdrbo, Hudak, Anthony, & Douglas, 2011). As this paper continues, it will discuss several key areas that must come together to support specialized electronic healthcare information systems. These areas include the potential impact of quality measures for the use of health information technology on patient care, the pros and cons for the use of best-of-breed versus integrated health information technology solutions, the two quality measures that would benefit nurses who have a voice in the selection of an electronic clinical system, and the advantages for the integration of data from pharmacy, laboratory, and radiology information systems with the electronic patient record. In addition, it will explain why the Leapfrog Group recommends the use of computerized provider order entry, examine the factors that impact the management of patient flow in hospitals, and consider at least three factors that promote the adoption of clinical information systems by nurses.

There is an array of healthcare information systems currently in use throughout the United States to manage all aspects of the patient care and business processes as they relate to healthcare. These healthcare information systems typically consist of multiple programs to track and manage the financial and patient care data. A system that is appropriately designed will consist of an interface that will allow for the communication and ease of transfer of data and information between systems.

An effective clinical documentation system should facilitate workflow and not dictate the process, it must also be nimble enough to allow for customization at the local level to facilitate workflow, incorporate new knowledge and monitor regulatory compliance. (Hall et al., 2013, p. 419–426).

At the selection stage of a system, the consumer must consider what is suitable to meet its institutional or departmental needs. The best-of-breed and integrated solutions are two known approaches in the selection of these systems. The best-of-breed approach is more specific in focusing on meeting needs on a departmental level. This will also usually require an integrated interface to allow for collaboration with the institutional system. On the other side, the integrated approach is a collection of systems that have already been interfaced at its inception but may not be the best of breed. There is also an enterprise system that is integrated to satisfy the needs and demands of an institution as a whole.

THE PHYSICIAN QUALITY REPORT INITIATIVE (PQRI)

Nurses and healthcare providers involved in the selection of health information technology (HIT) should be aware of the national quality initiative for HIT. The Physician Quality Report Initiative (PQRI) is one of these measures. The providers involved in the process of choosing these systems must also be mindful of its organizational demands and possess the necessary knowledge to assess vendor systems. The PQRI initiative came into play in 2006 as a part of a healthcare act. It came about due to the history of the American healthcare system being notorious for rewarding poor care rather than quality of care. The PQRI, an evidenced-base quality measure, allows for around a 2% reimbursement incentive to Medicare-authorized providers who voluntarily participate in the program. The program also includes information in regards to electronic health records (EHR).

Electronic health records are subject to a certification process. This process is completed through a private nonprofit organization called the Certification Commission for Healthcare Information Technology (CCHIT). This organization provides two certifications to ensure EHR interoperability for various ambulatory and inpatient care settings. Other certification organizations are aimed at evaluating the satisfaction of the meaningful use requirements. These certifying bodies are expected to grow in the near future.

Due to the cost of investment into these systems, it is only sensible to utilize research-based tools in assisting in the decision-making process. There are several research companies and nonprofit organizations that provide this information. Some are even free of charge. All the departments contained in a healthcare institution require specialized information needs. Although there is a need for a specialized focus, there are two common needs that are shared by all: access to a patient's electronic record and the ability to bill for services rendered through the financial management department. In the selection of a specialized health information system, best-of-breed or an integrated enterprise solution must be weighed into consideration.

ADMISSION, DISCHARGE, AND TRANSFER (ADT) SYSTEM

One of the very first information systems used in healthcare is the admission, discharge, and transfer (ADT) system, which serves as the foundation for the financial and business aspect of hospital systems. ADT systems continue to be a commonly integrated feature. This system collects demographic information and tracks patient interactions for ease of locating patients. These information technology systems, according to Hall and colleagues (Hall, et al 2013)

> [c]ould also include a clinical database or data repository where patterns are detected, comparative effectiveness [is] made between different treatment decisions, and outcome [is] measured to develop evidence-based guidelines. Furthermore, the data repository may place the power of evidence and research at the patient's bedside and into the hands of clinicians and organizational leaders. As a result, this can potentially allow for quality improvement teams and clinicians to be granted appropriate and secure access to answer various care delivery and outcome questions. (p. 419–426)

Since these systems continue to interoperate with ancillary departments, such as the lab, it is vital for these systems to be updated and checked on a regular basis. A secondary part to this foundation is the financial system. This system manages financial interactions as well as collects the fiscal data necessary to manage an institution. Since these systems are considered crucial to the existence of organizations, they are termed as mission critical. The financial systems allow for greater revenue collection and increase timely reimbursements and reduction of third-party payment denials. Many healthcare organizations are facing issues with outdated systems and how to get these systems to communicate with the clinical side of information systems. Some of these systems no longer meet the current regulatory demands. To avert the cumbersome job of building multiple interfaces to integrate these systems, some institutions have opted to purchase a very costly enterprise system. Some level of integration between the financial and the ADT system is necessary to effectively collect data for process improvements and for more efficient billing processes. Healthcare agencies face many challenges in their attempt to run as successful businesses while meeting regulatory and payment requirements. Also, these agencies want to be able to bill without being accused of fraudulent activity. The Center for Medicare and Medicaid (CMS) has programs in place to assess for false claims.

ELECTRONIC MEDICATION ADMINISTRATION RECORD (eMAR)

Clinical information systems encompass a large network of integrated and interoperable patient care information systems. Ancillary departments, such as pharmacy, radiology, and laboratory are the components that comprise the core information system. The electronic medication administration record (eMAR) and the positive patient identifier system (PPID) are also included in the makeup of clinical information systems. The PPID also includes the bar-coded medication administration system. PPID is an electronic documentation of medication administration which includes bar coded wrist bands for patients' identification and bar-coded medications. It also provides an internal check that alerts nurses to potential medication errors (Husting & Cintron, 2003). The vendors of clinical information systems are constantly striving to improve the performance and quality of their products. This activity provides the organizations serviced by the vendors with the competitive edge in optimizing service quality and improving efficiency and effectiveness, especially given the financial investments involved in evaluation of the effectiveness of technology (Adbrbo et al., 2011). It may be necessary for upgraded or more improved versions of their products to satisfy any effectiveness gaps.

PICTURE ARCHIVING AND COMMUNICATION SYSTEM (PACS)

For several decades, in many large and small healthcare systems throughout the country, laboratory, radiology, and pharmacy systems have been in place to store, track and view clinical data. One of the earliest radiology systems that is still in place in many institutions is the picture archiving and communication system (PACS). This type of information and communication technology enables biomedical knowledge, such as digital radiology images, to be rapidly disseminated. (Kaufman, Roberts, Merill, Lai, & Bakken, 2006). These three ancillary information systems provide a foundation for other clinical systems (Sewell & Thede, 2013).

There are many formats and applications available to perform clinical documentation. It is a known fact that an efficient documentation system would give the user an opportunity to accomplish the changes necessary to meet future challenges and provide real-time actionable information (Hall et al., 2013). These systems are designed to flag abnormal values. This is usually achieved by highlighting these values in a different color than the normal or expected value. It eliminates the need to rummage through a paper chart to locate this vital and potentially lifesaving information.

Assessment documentation can be systematically depicted by other displays such as graphs that would demonstrate trends. The best systems would have very little need for free text data entry with a reiteration that it is imperative that information technology infrastructure must be more robust and redesigned to be more than a substitute for paper documentation (Hall et al., 2013). These systems will work well when the healthcare providers that use the systems are directly involved in the implementation process.

Some different information systems utilize a nursing process approach as the framework. This typically supports a more seamless clinical workflow. It should also institute a means for accessing up-to-date literature, research, hospital policies, and procedures. Also important in clinical documentation systems is the ability to allow for nurses and providers to see the big picture by aggregating data. This facilitates the ease of data retrieval and interpretation for the determination of best practices.

COMPUTERIZED PROVIDER ORDER ENTRY (CPOE)

Highly supported by the Leapfrog Group to improve patient safety and quality is the use of the computerized provider order entry (CPOE). It allows for providers to enter orders by selecting patients and also serves at abating multi-million-dollar preventable adverse medication errors. It increases efficiency because the order is immediately sent to the appropriate department. In addition, it allows for ease of capturing financial information for billing and tracking purposes. Another attribute to the CPOE is e-prescribing. This method of ordering medications improves quality care because all medication orders are first checked against the clinical decision support system information. The clinical decision support system serves as an up-to-date database to support prescribers in their clinical decision making and alert potential drug allergies and incompatibilities. The CPOE also makes the medication administration process safer by reducing the risk of error. Prior to the computerized era of medication administration, the hand-written process consisted of three steps: the written doctor's order, the pharmacist's verification and dispensing of the order, and the nurse's administration and documentation of such order. This process is consolidated with the use of electronic medication administration records (eMARs). eMARs document the entire multidisciplinary process involved in medication use. It serves as a guide to nurses that follows the six rights of medication administration. The Joint Commission first issued a recommendation for accurately identifying patients in 2003 (Sewell & Thede, 2013). It schedules medication administration times, queues nurses into order discrepancies, flags for expiring orders, and facilitates the highest level of safe medication delivery. This safety in delivery is potentiated by the use of the PPID-barcoded bracelets, discussed earlier. eMars allow for a closed-loop, safe medication administration method. This method uses a barcode scanner, often an active or passive radio frequency identifier (RFID) utilizing a handheld or laptop scanning device.

Multiple research studies have been conducted and are in support of a CPOE system. On the other hand, some nurses find this impeding to perform their medication administration. It is important for nurses to understand the potential detrimental and lethal effects of these workarounds. One study that is discussed by Sewell and Thede (2013) reveals seven types of process workarounds as follows: scanning the medication without verifying the medication list, drug name, and dose; physicians not verifying the eMar current medication list, resulting in additional medication given to the patient; administering the medication without reviewing the parameters for administration; bypassing the policy for a check by a second provider or the second nurse confirms without verifying the medication; administering medications without reviewing new medication orders; administering medications without scanning the patient's barcode to confirm the patient's identification; and administering the medication without scanning the medication barcode to confirm the correct medication, dose, and time. Administrators must remain keen to the workarounds that occur in their departments and implement investigative measures to deter these unsafe medication administration behaviors.

Patient flow continues to be a long-standing issue at healthcare facilities. It must be recognized and addressed to preserve a safe and efficient patient care environment. The issues attributed to patient flow are multifaceted but fall back to the basic principle of supply and demand. Staffing, supplies, and resources are all budgeted for average to low hospital census, when in retrospect most institutions are performing at a higher level. This creates a disparity between hospital economics and efficiency. Patient flow problems usually start at the emergency room, especially during the peak flu season when the usual population of chronically ill patients are disproportionately outnumbered by the rise in patients presenting as acutely ill with upper respiratory or flu-like symptoms. Sewell and Thede (2013) pointed out another Joint Commission recommendation that calls on hospitals to discover and minimize barriers to well-organized patient flow. This went into effect in 2005 and was in part based on a research study that found that overcrowding in emergency departments was a contributing factor in about one third of hospital sentinel events. This drove many hospitals to implement informatics bed management systems to ensure appropriate patient placement the first time around.

Most EMR systems also provide informatics solutions to track patient's locations and monitor the patient flow process. They act as visual aids to display beds, bed status, patient status, isolation issues, notification of need of ancillary departments, and equipment location. Sewell and Thede (2013) report on a study conducted on a hospital in Delaware that showed significant improvement in patient flow with the implementation of a specific tracking tools. The total length of stay in the ED for patients improved and the number of patients left without being seen decreased, which led to greater turnaround and efficiency and ultimately resulted in raised patient volume.

VOICE COMMUNICATION SYSTEMS

Another piece of technology currently being used in healthcare settings is voice communication systems. These systems facilitate a more efficient exchange of information by various healthcare disciplines. An example of this technology is the Vocera system that I have used in my area of work. This type of system, although not integrated with clinical systems, enhances workflow productivity. The Vocera system is a wireless voice recognition communication and location device that is lightweight and portable. It can be clipped to your scrub top or blouse. Research studies on the Vocera support positive patient and departmental outcomes that result in financial benefits in the tens of thousands. Suggestions have been made that the Vocera system and similar voice-over-Internet protocol technologies are now considered outdated in the healthcare arena. Current technologies include smartphones. These devices are the latest in voice communication devices. They allow for ease of data encryption, are easily disinfected, have anti-theft capabilities, and, most importantly, are easily integrated with EMR. Smart phone technologies are slowly driving overhead paging systems and pagers to extinction.

Clinical pathways are made more feasible by information systems. They have been developed through research and synthesis of these research findings. These pathways are structurally constructed to give way to multidisciplinary access and documentation and define a specific clinical goal within specific time frame parameters. Point of care interventions should allow for access to clinical information systems at that time or at a point where the nurse has an opportunity to sit and reflect through documentation on that intervention. According to Sewell and Thede (2013), nurses' attitudes are often shaped by the ease and/or difficulty in use. It has been noted that nurses tend to argue the use of computers in healthcare, stating that they do not follow a natural, holistic, and humanistic approach as nursing should, and that computers are complex devices to work with. These devices are often attached to heavy, bulky carts that may be cumbersome to maneuver and these carts may have wheels that get stuck or fall off. Studies have concluded that the user profile, including age, marital status, education, type of facility, job title, computer science education and experience, duration of computer use, and environment, are important variables that significantly affected the development of nurses' positive attitudes toward computers (Kay, 2011, pp. 127–128).

With the rapidly changing complex healthcare environment, use of advanced health information technology is an essential necessity. Health information technology (HIT) has been used to enhance and improve care and outcomes for older adults in a growing program directed by current strategic policies in line with the Health Information Technology for Economic and Clinical Health (HITECH) Act (Blumenthal, 2010; Institute of Medicine, 2011). Quality continues to be the driving force that demands the most up-to-date information technology systems. The advantages and disadvantages of best-of-breed systems versus integrated enterprise solutions that were outlined in this paper need to always be considered when selecting a specialized electronic healthcare information system.

References

Abdrbo, A., Hudak, C., Anthony, M., & Douglas, S. (2011). Information systems use, benefits, and satisfaction among Ohio RNs. *Computers, Informatics, Nursing, 29*(1), 59–65.

American Medical Association. (2013). *Patient confidentiality*. Retrieved from https://journalofethics.ama-assn.org/taxonomy/confidentialitypatient-privacy?page=2

Automatic identification and data capture market 2018 global analysis, opportunities and forecast to 2026. Retrieved from https://www.marketwatch.com/press-release/automatic-identification-and-data-capture-market-2018-global-analysis-opportunities-and-forecast-to-2026-2018-11-15

Azari, A., Janeja, V. P., Mohseni, A. (2012). Predicting hospital length of stay (PHLOS): A multi-tiered data mining approach. Data Mining Workshops (ICDMW), IEEE 12th International Conference, Brussels, Belgium Belgium, ISBN: 978-1-4673-5164-5 pp: 17-24, http://doi.ieeecomputersociety.org/10.1109/ICDMW.2012.69

Blumenthal D. Launching HITECH. New England Journal of Medicine. 2010;362(5):382–385. [PubMed]

Busch, R (2008). Electronic Health Records: An Audit and Internal Control Guide Publisher: John Wiley & Sons, ISBN: 9780470258200. https://www.oreilly.com/library/view/electronic-health-records/9780470258200/

Cain, C., & Haque, S. (2008). Organizational workflow and its impact on work quality. In *patient safety and quality: An evidence-based handbook for nurses* (Chapter 3). Hughes RG, editor.

Rockville (MD): Agency for Healthcare Research and Quality (US). Retrieved from https://www.ncbi.nlm.nih.gov/books/NBK2638/

Chaiken, B. P. (2011). *Transforming health care through improved clinician workflows*. Sacramento, CA iHealth Beat.

Cheswick, W. (2003). *Firewalls and Internet security*. India: Pearson.

Croskerry, P., & Cosby, K. S. (2009). Patient safety in emergency medicine. Philadelphia, PA: Lippincott Williams & Wilkins.

Elsevier-SimChart (2017). Retrieved from https://web.archive.org/web/20130118104219/http://elsevieradvantage.com/article.jsp?pageid=11640

Finney, M. A., McHugh, C. W., Grenfell, I. C., Riley, K. L., & Short, K. (2011) A simulation of probabilistic wildfire risk components for the continental United States., *Stochastic Environmental Research And Risk Assessment Journal*, 25, 973–1000. Retrieved from https://www.fs.fed.us/rm/pubs_other/rmrs_2011_finney_m002.pdfGarrett, P. & Seidman, J. (2011). *EMR vs EHR—What is the difference?* Retrieved from https://www.healthit.gov/buzz-blog/electronic-health-and-medical-records/emr-vs-ehr-difference

Garrett, P., & Seidman, J. (2011) EMR vs EHR. What is the difference? Health IT Buzz health. Retrieved from www.healthit.gov/buzz.blogg/electronic-health-and-medical-records/emr-vs-ehr-difference/ on October 3 2013

Hall, P., Poole, R., & Hall, C. (2013). Bridging the gaps in supportive information systems. *Home Healthcare Nurse*, 31(8), 419–426. Retrieved from https://books.google.com/books?id=KmxLAAAAMAAJ&pg=RA11-PR3&lpg=RA11-PR3&dq=Hall,+P.,+Poole,+R.,+%26+Hall,+C.+(2013).&source=bl&ots=VonAuxF6tu&sig=9ruL7RzyxhERCPR8IEIXIlHcToA&hl=en&sa=X&ved=2ahUKEwipy9uayrTfAhWqT98KHU-FCDcQ6AEwAX0ECAUQAQ#v=onepage&q=Hall%2C%20P.%2C%20Poole%2C%20R.%2C%20%26%20Hall%2C%20C.%20(2013).&f=false

Health IT. (n.d.). Putting the "I" in health IT. Retrieved from http://www.healthit.gov/patients-families/health-it-makes-health-care-convenient

Hebda, T., & Czar, P. (2009). *Handbook of informatics for nurses and healthcare professionals* (5th ed.). Upper Saddle River, NJ: Pearson.

Hebda, T., & Czar, P. (2012). *Handbook of informatics for nurses & healthcare professionals* (5th ed.). Boston, MA: Pearson.

Husting, P., & Cintron, L. (2003). Healthcare information systems: Education lessons learned. *Journal for Nurses in Staff Development*, 19(5), 249–253.

Institute of Medicine. The future of nursing: Leading change, advancing health. 2010 Retrieved: 2012, Retrieved fromhttp://books.nap.edu/openbook.php?record_id=12956&page=R1.

Kaufman, D., Roberts, D., Merrill, J., Lai, T. Y., & Bakken, S. (2006). Applying an evaluation framework for health information system design, development, implementation. *Nursing Research*, 55(2), 37–42.

Kaya, N. (2011). Factors affecting nurses' attitudes toward computers in healthcare. *Computers, Informatics, Nursing*, 29(2), 121–129. http://nursing-informatics.com/niassess/00024665-201102000-00009.pdfHanks, R. G. (2010). Development and testing of an instrument to measure protective nursing advocacy. *Nurse Ethics*, 17(2), 255.

Kurtz, G. (2003). EMR confidentiality and information security. *Journal of Healthcare Information Management*, 17(3). Retrieved from http://europepmc.org/abstract/med/12858596

Lippincott Williams & Wilkins (2012). *Electronic Health Record (EHR) Learning Tool to Help Future Nurses Prepare for New Practice Requirements. Retrieved from* https://wolterskluwer.com/company/newsroom/news/health/2012/07/lippincott-williams--wilkins-launches-electronic-health-record-ehr-learning-tool-to-help-future-nurses-prepare-for-new-practice-requirements.html

Maheu, M. M., Whitten, P., & Allen, A. (2001). *Jossey-Bass health series. E-health, telehealth, and telemedicine: A guide to start-up and success.* San Francisco, CA, US: Jossey-Bass.

McAfee, A. (2006). Enterprise 2.0: The dawn of emergent collaboration. *MIT Sloan Management Review, 47*(3), 21–28.

National Academy of Sciences. (2013). *Sharing clinical research data: Workshop summary.* Retrieved from https://www.nap.edu/read/18267/chapter/1

Norris, A. C. (2002). Essentials of telemedicine and telecare. West Sussex, UK: Wiley.

Olmeda, C. J. (2000). Information technology in systems of care. Delfin Press.

Orlovsky, C. (2011). The endless nursing benefits of electronic medical records. *Nurse Zone.* Retrieved from https://susiecookhc.wordpress.com/2011/04/25/endless-nursing-benefits-of-electronic-medical-records-emr/

Office of the National Coordinator for Health Information Technology (2013). Enabling Health Information Exchange to Support Community Goals. *A Learning Guide.* p. 1. Retrieved from https://www.healthit.gov/sites/default/files/onc-beacon-lg4-clinical-transformation-via-hit.pdf

Saba V. K., Taylor SL.(2007). Moving past theory: use of a standardized, coded nursing terminology to enhance nursing visibility. *Computers, Informatics, Nursing* 25(6):324–31.

Saba, V., & McCormick, K. (2011). *Essentials of nursing informatics.* (5th ed.) New York, NY: McGraw-Hill.

Savage, G. T., & Ford, E. W. (2008). *Patient safety and health care management.* Bingley, UK: Emerald Group.

Schwirian, P. M. (2013). Informatics and the future of nursing: Harnessing the power of standardized nursing terminology. *Health Informatics, 39*(5), 20–24.

Sewell, J., & Thede, L. (2013). Informatics and nursing: Opportunities and challenges (4th ed.). Philadelphia, PA: Lippincott Williams Wilkins.

Shoniregun, C. A., & Dube, K. (2010). Electronic healthcare information security. Dublin, Ireland: Springer.

Silow-Carroll, S., Edward S. J. N., & Rodin, D. (2012). Using electronic health records to improve quality and efficiency: The experiences of leading hospitals. Issue Brief (Commonw Fund). 2012 Jul, 17: 1–40.Retrieved from https://www.ncbi.nlm.nih.gov/pubmed/22826903

Simpson, R. L. (2006). Ethics and information technology: How nurses balance when integrity and trust are at stake. *Nursing Administration Quarterly, 30*(1), 82–87.

Singer, Jonathan B. (2009). The Role and Regulations for Technology in Social Work Practice and E-Therapy: Social Work 2.0. New York, U.S.A.: Oxford University Press.

Tan, J., & Payton, F. C. (2012). *Adaptive health management information systems: Concepts, cases, and practical applications.* London, UK: Jones & Bartlett.

Thede, L., Schwiran, P., (2011) "Informatics: The Standardized Nursing Terminologies: A National Survey of Nurses' Experiences and Attitudes" OJIN: The Online Journal of Issues in Nursing Vol. 16 No. 2.

Thede, L., Schwirian, P., (2015) "Informatics: The Standardized Nursing Terminologies: A National Survey of Nurses' Experience and Attitudes—SURVEY II: Evaluation of Standardized Nursing Terminologies" *The Online Journal of Issues in Nursing: The Online Journal of Issues in Nursing* Vol. 21 No. 1., http://ojin.nursingworld.org/MainMenuCategories/ANAMarketplace/ANAPeriodicals/OJIN/Columns/Informatics/Survey-II-Evaluation-of-Standardized-Nursing-Terminologies.html#Schwirian11

Triggle, N. (2013, April 1). NHS structure changes come into force. *BBC News*. Retrieved from http://www.bbc.co.uk/news/health-21964568

U. S. Department of Health and Human Services. (2003). *Summary of the HIPAA Privacy Rule*. Retrieved from https://www.hhs.gov/hipaa/for-professionals/privacy/laws-regulations/index.html

Whittenburg, L. (2010). Workflow viewpoints: Analysis of nursing workflow documentation. *Journal of Healthcare Information Management*, 24(3):71–5.

Wikipedia (2018). *Microchip implant*. Retrieved from https://en.wikipedia.org/wiki/Microchip_implant_%28human%29

CHAPTER 12

Health Information Confidentiality, Security, and Integrity

CHAPTER HIGHLIGHTS

This chapter discusses the following:

- How the technology boom has increased the risk of many sources being threatened, leading the components of the system to be open to vulnerabilities
- How private institutions and the government have implemented new security measures to protect the healthcare information of its consumers to prevent threats of jeopardizing the confidentiality and information integrity of a system and high publicized medical breaches

WITH THE INCREASED use of information technology and the new mandate by the American Recovery and Reinvestment Act, approved by President Obama and requiring all hospitals to adopt electronic health records by 2014, there has been an increase threat to information security and confidentiality (Hebda & Czar 2009). In fact, 40% of medical data breaches have involved the usage of portable devices such as laptops or hard drives. It's indeed an outrageously high statistic and could have been alleviated if simple measures had been taken—it is not acceptable in today's hi-tech environment (Schultz, 2012). The technology boom has increased the risk of many sources being threatened, leading the components of the system to be open to vulnerabilities. This has led the government to implement strict guidelines in efforts to protect health records for effective client care. Other security measures such as encryption, work design, biometrics, and the regulation of limiting access to electronic health records are being employed to lower the incidence of unsecure health records. With the outrageously high incidents of healthcare breaches and the awareness and the emergence of new technologies to reinvent the design of the existing healthcare system, the improvement of information security and confidentiality will increase.

SYSTEM THREATS

Every day, people unconsciously participate in activities on their personal computers that compromise their security, allowing their computers to be prone to hackers, terrorists, viruses, etc. Hebda & Czar (2009) has compiled a list that notes the top 10 security threats, ranging from social networks and wireless networks. These threats can lead to a list of issues such as identity theft, monetary loss, and violations to confidentiality and information integrity, especially in the healthcare delivery system. There is a direct relationship between the possible threats of a system (e.g., hackers, terrorist) and vulnerabilities of a system/network. Vulnerabilities in regards to the procedures, design, implementation, or internal control could result in a security breach or violation of the system's policy. Therefore, the increase in system threats will also increase vulnerability, allowing for unsecure sites, malicious software, worms, etc. With threats jeopardizing the confidentiality and information integrity of a system and highly publicized medical breaches, the government has implemented new security measures to protect the healthcare information of its consumers (Hebda & Czar, 2009).

SURVEILLANCE MEASURES

Different surveillance measures have been introduced to protect the security of information and computer systems. These mechanisms range from simple passwords, establishing firewalls and installing antivirus and spyware to the process of authentication. Passwords are utilized by common people every day as well as by many agencies. Although passwords can provide some protection from unauthorized individuals opening documents/computer systems, they are an extremely weak security measure. They have many disadvantages because they can be guessed by a person or by a program. Other security measures that can hold importance include biometrics. For example, an employee would be able to use a unique biological trait such as a fingerprint or voice to retrieve information (Czar & Hebda, 2009). Unlike passwords, this type of authentication remains with the individual and cannot be stolen or lost. This will reduce the need of the healthcare agency to allocate time to reset passwords. With regards to work design, it is critical that computers are set up and arranged within the hospital to prevent threats to security. Also, proper education must be provided to healthcare providers to prevent breaches and violation of security. It is crucial that these simple security measures are being implemented within the system's security to help manage and operate its protection.

With all the possible dangers of the system, the government has implemented new policies and procedures for healthcare agencies' compliance to reduce the incidents of the violations of privacy and confidentiality. This decision has led the Joint Commission to enforce the government mandate, the Health Insurance Portability Act (HIPAA), in 1996. The new objective of the system rules is to safeguard the integrity and security of clients' information. Therefore, it is the agency's or the hospital's policy to integrate different measures such as encryption to assist with this government mandate. To further stress the importance of HIPAA, if the agency does not meet the set requirements, they may face extreme financial penalties. In fact, the Health Information Technology for Economic and Clinical Health Act (HITECH) created more rigorous rules for any form of disclosure, privacy monitoring, and the usage of medical information for marketing.

> Corporate misconduct is a classic justification for expending societal resources to hold a company accountable and deter other companies from engaging in similar, harmful conduct. However, company data on consumers and clients may be compromised in situations involving no corporate

misconduct. In fact, in many situations the hacker is the primary culprit. The theft of personal information causes minimal harm to consumers, while the business-the putative defendant-suffers far greater costs associated with a breach. Prevention is costly and difficult, and predicting which companies will be hacked, as well as the means by which it will occur, is next to impossible. (Marian & Riedy, 2016, p. 3).

ENCRYPTION

New security measures such as encryption have been implemented to safeguard health information. According to the Competitive Enterprise Institute, encryption is defined as the usage of difficult math to encode the text of a document into a code. For one to understand the text and return the document to "plain text," one must have a key. Encryption allows authorized users to access healthcare information, thus preventing hackers from accessing important client data. However, encryption doesn't protect employees or nurse managers from abusing their powers of reviewing or accessing information (Singleton, 2011).

SPECIFIC CASE SCENARIOS AS SEEN FROM STUDENTS' PERSPECTIVES

Case Study #1: Patient Information and HIPAA

"In the course of your daily activities at work, your nurse coordinator tells you he loaded a copy of the PowerPoint program he uses on his home office Mac onto one of the unit computers so that he could work on projects at both locations. Your institution has a well-publicized policy against the use of unauthorized, unlicensed software copies." As a staff nurse, what should you do? (Hebda & Czar, 2009).

As a staff nurse, I would follow the chain of commands and report this incident to the right individual. The nurse manager working on a PP at home and work gives hackers a higher chance of invading the privacy of the patients and gives viruses a chance to attack the computer. Also, the agency should host employee compliance programs or provide information security manuals to emphasize this misdemeanor (Singleton, 2001). Perhaps one of the hindrances of using Macs at healthcare facilities is not the potential threat of unauthorized usage from outsiders, but from insiders also. Thus, access of confidential information should be strictly limited to a need-to-know basis, where the information can only be accessed under a particular condition or event. In this way, an audit trail will be created every time the employee accesses the Mac for information. Another way of monitoring access is by setting limits for every level of personnel based on defining roles or scopes of practice. Therefore, "user classes" should be established to provide different privileges. Direct care providers will then be able to acquire information about their clients without abusing sensitive healthcare information.

In conclusion, it is very important to implement these new security measures because healthcare professionals are now facing the consequences associated with the violations mandated by the Health Insurance and Portability Act (HIPAA). The American Recovery and Reinvestment Act also creates more risk of unsecure information being released. Therefore, it is vital that these security measures are being adopted. Utilizing biometric measures for authentication is expected to replace the mundane use of a password. Biometric authentication helps organizations be in compliance with state and federal regulations; it also reduces the time spent resetting passwords. The particular healthcare agency utilizes training programs to ensure that authorized users are not abusing their powers and possibly altering healthcare information. The levels of access should be centered around the healthcare provider scope of practice. The healthcare provider should only have access to client information, in which he or she is an active member of the healthcare team. With the greater concern, awareness, and commitment in protecting client's pertinent healthcare information, the future for information security and confidentiality is moving into a better direction.

Case Study #2: Informatics and Patient Care

As a result of new and emerging technology and changing consumer expectations, healthcare will inevitably transition to a more person- and family-centric health system requiring the interoperability of a broad array of health solutions from traditional resources, including clinicians and hospitals, to the internet of things (Ommaya, Cipriano, Hoyt, Horvath, Tang, Paz, DeFrancesco, Hingle, Butler and Sinsky, 2018. p. 1)

Furthering the use of informatics in the nursing practice setting would thus be in full consonance with the mission and values of the nursing profession. The purpose of this case study is to consider the case of a patient (hereafter referred to as "Amos") who has arrived in the emergency department with shortness of breath and is complaining of chest pain, and to discuss the positive effects which the use of healthcare informatics can have on the efficiency, safety, and quality of nursing care delivered to Amos. Specific aspects of the situation that will be considered include but are not limited to electronic health records (EHRs), decision support systems, and inter-professional collaboration. To start with, if Amos has a comprehensive EHR, then healthcare professionals can save a great deal of time in retrieving and analyzing the patient's medical history. In the specific situation under consideration, it is worth noting that Amos has shown up to the emergency room, and he is short of breath—meaning that the situation could turn urgent and that full-scale communication with the patient may be difficult. This is exactly the sort of situation in which an efficient way of getting up to date with the patient's health status may prove crucial. EHR technology can fulfill this function and provides healthcare professionals with timely and comprehensive empirical knowledge. EHR technology often raises ethical questions; for example, the freedom of information it implies may threaten the value of patient confidentiality and healthcare professionals, in their zeal to assist the patient, may be susceptible to overstepping certain boundaries in this regard. However, the benefits to efficiency conferred by EHR are indisputable.

In addition, the use of EHR technology can enhance the safety of the care delivered to Amos as well. If Amos is presently on any medications or has any allergies, conditions, etc. that are contraindicated with certain treatment options, this will be immediately clear to the healthcare professionals at hand. Again, the nature of the situation is such that in-depth communication with the patient may not be possible and retrieving information with the assistance of EHR may be the only way to adequately ensure that the patient would not suffer from any adverse reactions to the chosen treatment strategy.

From the basis of the patient's manifest condition and the information provided by the EHR, nurses can proceed to make assessments and diagnoses for Amos, and at this point, healthcare informatics could play the role of providing clinical decision support. In the context of a culture of technology in which all healthcare professionals have vast stores of empirical information and knowledge available at their fingertips, the nursing care delivered to Amos will be as scientifically sound and as thorough as possible. Also, it is worth reiterating that the issue is not only knowledge, but also speed and timeliness; informatics can assist not only with delivering relevant information, but also with processing and delivering that information precisely when it is needed. This is especially pertinent for patients such as Amos who is experiencing a health emergency.

Healthcare informatics cannot only assist with efficiently retrieving both Amos's personal health information and information relevant to pursuing treatment, it can also assist with analyzing the interface between these sets of information. For example, if an adequate information system is in place, then nurses may be able to use technology to automatically identify links between certain symptoms, certain diagnoses, and certain treatment strategies. There is admittedly a danger involved, here: If nurses become too reliant on such technologies, they may "lose their instincts," so to speak, and neglect more subjective modes of nursing knowledge (Zander, 2008). Even so, in the case of Amos, the most important thing is to effectively address the immediate present symptoms, and informatics can help nurses efficiently come to a workable understanding of the patient's situation. This understanding can be both deepened and complemented once the patient's condition has stabilized.

Thus far, this case study has focused on the nurse being able to obtain information from inanimate records, databases, and the like. However, healthcare informatics can catalyze not only the retrieval and analysis of information, but also the *communication* of information between various healthcare professionals. In the case of patient Amos, it may not be immediately clear to nurses exactly what service the patient needs provided—and, consequently, which specific healthcare professionals need to be involved in his case. For example, perhaps Amos needs medication; perhaps he needs rest; perhaps he needs someone with whom to talk; perhaps he needs surgery in the very near future. If only paper records are available, then the number of professionals who could retrieve information about Amos will be necessarily limited; but with EHR, no such limits exist. Instead of needing to waste time repeating the same "story" to every new healthcare professional consulted, the relevant data and information can be made available to all potentially relevant professionals from the beginning.

The implications of this activity for communication can be better understood with reference to McDaniel, Lanham, and Anderson's (2009) concept of a complex adaptive system in which the various relevant parties are related to each other in nonlinear ways. Whereas a normal system, undergirded by pen-and-paper information records, could be understood as facilitating linear, or "arithmetic," communication, a complex adaptive system undergirded by an electronic information network could be understood as facilitating exponential—or geometric—communication. In short, the possible collaborations between various healthcare professionals and flows of skills and knowledge increase dramatically when everyone is connected by virtue of a nonlinear complex adaptive system. This will, of course, have positive consequences on the quality of care ultimately delivered to Amos, because this care will be maximally streamlined.

Finally, once healthcare professionals have completed delivering care to Amos, healthcare informatics can also help ensure adequate discharge of the patient in such a way that the risk of patient re-admission is minimized. For example, if it is determined that the patient should begin taking a certain medication, then technology can be used to set up a schedule and a system of reminders to help Amos comply with the medication protocol. As another example, Amos's immediate symptoms seem to indicate some sort of heart condition, and such conditions are often chronic. In such a situation, the hospital may determine that Jonah should follow up with a community nurse to develop a lifestyle that will prevent Jonah from experiencing any emergency in the future. This would require coordination not only between different healthcare professionals, but healthcare professionals working in different settings. By being able to simultaneously consult Amos's EHR, professionals from both the hospital and the community setting may be able to work together to optimize Amos's health. Furthermore, the patient himself would need to be actively included in any such plan, and healthcare informatics can facilitate this inclusion as "regression analyses has shown factors which shape the expected outcomes of personal Internet use during work, such as a generalized positive perception of the utility of the Internet, routinized use of computers, job commitment, and organizational restrictions on computer use, are very significant predictors of the computer use behavior at work" (Smith et al., 2011, p.1).

In summary, this case study has reviewed various ways in which healthcare informatics could assist with delivering high-quality care to a patient such as Amos.

One of the fundamental technologies discussed was the EHR; this would help healthcare professionals efficiently retrieve and analyze information regarding the patient. However, this is only the beginning; with this information in hand, nurses can both match the information against the best clinical knowledge available and communicate this information simultaneously to all other healthcare professionals involved in the patient's case. Safety of care is improved due to the ability to ensure that chosen treatment strategies are not in any way contraindicated; quality of care is improved due to the streamlining and patient centeredness provided by inter-professional collaboration, and efficiency of care is improved all around. On the basis of this hypothetical case study, it should be clear that healthcare informatics has a huge potential to further the mission and vision of the nursing profession. There is some need for ethical and epistemological caution with respect to the proliferation of technology, but as long as this caution is maintained, the potential of healthcare informatics should surely be pursued.

Case Study #3: Legal and Ethical Issues

Electronic medical records (EMRs) strongly promote the free flow of information, and this can have significant positive effects on values such as the quality and efficiency of healthcare. However, insofar as the value of confidentiality is meant precisely to *restrict* the flow of information, it can be suggested that the proliferation of EMRs implies certain risks for the preservation of confidentiality. The purpose of this case study is to assess three aspects of a scenario about this dilemma involving the registered nurse James. In the first aspect, James's mother is admitted to his unit; in the second, James's unit clerk has access to the mother's EMR; and in the third, James's coworker (Mary) is assigned (as a patient) to the care of another staff nurse in the unit. The question to be explored in the first and third aspects is whether it would be appropriate for James to access the EMRs of his mother or coworker; and in the second, the question is whether it would be appropriate for the unit clerk to access the mother's EMR.

To start, it is worth noting that what all three aspects of this scenario have in common is that there is personal interest involved. In the two aspects involving James himself, he has a personal connection with the other person. Moreover, in the aspect involving the unit clerk, it is presumable that the unit clerk has an indirect personal interest in James's mother because, otherwise, the question of appropriateness wouldn't even come up, since the unit clerk would have no desire to go beyond standard protocol in examining EMRs. The real question in this scenario seems to be "Is it appropriate for a nurse (or unit clerk) who is authorized to see a patient's EMR to do so on the basis of personal interest as opposed to professional necessity?" If James (or the unit clerk) needed to see his mother's or Mary's EMR as a standard part of simply doing his duty, then the whole scenario would be a nonissue (in fact, the only thinkable issue is that James, out a desire *not* to see the EMRs, may ask for reassignment). The real problem in this scenario is that James or the unit clerk may use their professional credentials to pursue personal interests by going beyond the bounds of professional duty. It can be seen that in this scenario, the presence of the unit clerk's aspect is superfluous because the ethics involved in the unit clerk's aspects and James's aspect of the scenario are exactly the same. Actually, the same ethical issue is present in *all three* aspects of the scenario; so, for the sake of simplicity, the remainder of this case study will focus only on the aspect of James and his mother under the assumption that whatever conclusion is reached for this aspect of the scenario will be applicable to all three aspects.

An important issue in this scenario would seem to be respect for autonomy; it is presumable that if James were to seek out his mother's EMR, he would be doing so either without her awareness or against her will because, in fact, there would nothing preventing her from freely sharing her information with her son if she chose to. Advocacy on behalf of the patient is enshrined in the ANA's (2001) Code of Ethics as one of the primary duties of the nurse, and this clearly implies not only respecting the autonomy of the patient, but also standing up for that autonomy in any and all circumstances. James has access to his mother's EMR, not in his capacity as son, but in his capacity of nurse; and, conversely, in this scenario James's mother must be understood not in terms of her role as mother, but rather in terms of her role of patient. The conclusion seems to follow from this analysis that James is entitled to no special prerogative because one of the patients in his ward happens to be his mother. In other words, he must stand up for the rights of his mother, and it would be unethical for him to pursue his personal interest as a son at the expense of his professional duty to engage in advocacy for the patient.

Again, if the mother wants to share her EMR with her son in her personal capacity as a mother, then it is presumable that no one would stop her. However, in his capacity as son, Kevin clearly wouldn't be able to access his mother's EMR without her knowledge or against her will; he would only be able to achieve such a feat in his capacity as nurse, and it is clearly unethical for a nurse to engage in such practices. It is unclear whether the mother would be aware of the dynamics involved in this scenario, given that "patients often either underestimate or overestimate the extent of confidentiality protections" and otherwise have some degree of confusion regarding the concept of confidentiality (Sankar, Moran, Merz, & Jones, 2003, p. 1 & 2). However, in his role as nurse, it would be James's duty not to take advantage of his mother's lack of clear knowledge, but rather to work toward ensuring that she adequately understands her rights.

To reiterate, the conclusions being drawn here with respect to James and his mother are also directly applicable to the aspects of James and Mary as well as the unit clerk and James's mother. This is because in both these aspects, the real issue is the conflation of personal and professional roles. Of course, it is likely that James's personal interest in Mary is of a lesser magnitude than his interest in his mother, and that the unit clerk's interest in James's mother may be rather fleeting compared to James's interest in either his mother or his coworker. However, in the present case study's reading of this scenario, it is the same ethical issue that instantiates all three aspects of this scenario, albeit with differential magnitudes, and therefore conclusions drawn from the greatest magnitude aspect will be applicable to the other aspects because analysis of the former (that is, the aspect of James and his mother) allows one to glean insight about the ethical issue in its purest form.

It is worth noting that one unclear point in the description of the scenario under consideration is that whether James has *access* to the EMRs of all the patients in his ward implies that he is also *authorized* to peruse those EMRs whenever he chooses and for whatever reason. For example, it is possible that his access is a result of the way the EMR system access is assigned, but he would need further credentials to make legitimate use of this access. This may be a case in which the evolution of the ethical doctrine of patient confidentiality is lagging behind technological innovations, which compromise the traditional understanding of that doctrine. In general, it would seem that just because any nurse *can* access the EMR of any patient does not mean that this *should* occur; and, in fact, nurses making widespread use of this privilege would almost certainly violate the doctrine of patient confidentiality.

Finally, even assuming that James is authorized as a professional to view his mother's EMR, the mother in her capacity as patient may have the right to explicitly request for a re-assignment such that her son will no longer have this authorization. This is due to the patient-centered and holistic nature of nursing practice: if there is reason to believe that a particular circumstance will cause significant psychosocial distress to the patient, then it is the duty of the nurse to do whatever is possible to ameliorate the causes of this distress (Kolcaba, 1994). The specific resolution to this sort of patient concern may differ across the three aspects of the scenario under consideration because the level of distress may be correlated with the closeness of the relationship. For example, James and his mother presumably have a close personal relationship; he and Mary, though, may have a relationship that is more cordial than personal (unless they happen to be, say, friends or lovers), and the relationship between the unit clerk and James's mother is only an indirect one. The hospital may need to exercise some case-by-case judgment in determining whether the patient's concern is reasonable given the nature of the relationship and whether the concern can be reasonably accommodated given the hospital's resources.

Case Study #4: Data Integrity

People go to hospitals because of illness. Some people fear hospitals because they do not know if going to one can be beneficial or costly; some have also had bad experiences with errors occurring during their care, which leads them to feel more comfortable avoiding care. On the other hand, most people want to feel safe and secure when entering a healthcare facility by trusting the healthcare team to bring them back to health and to promote health wellness. Nurses are a critical part of the healthcare team, and nursing informatics allows them to provide phenomenal care from the information collected and studies done to increase wellness.

Through the use of informatics, nurses can better ensure patient safety and wellness. Examples include the reduction of identification errors during procedures and medication administration (Hebda & Czar, 2005). Hebda states that "barcodes and radio frequency identification (RFID) are the dominant technologies for this" (Hebda et al, 2005, p. 17). This helps assure that we are entering the right information for the right patient. In this case study, the error could have been avoided if the nurse had scanned the patient identification bracelet to enter the information in her chart. In addition, if it was done in a different location, it would be helpful if the computer requested the patients' date of birth to enter the information in the right chart for the right patient.

Moreover, all data related to patients can be managed using a database application. This enables effective communication between interpersonal or intrapersonal healthcare providers for case management. It is also used by authorized personal from administrations or third parties in a less costly manner. The application of databases plays a very important role in providing safe and effective care to patients. Errors and mistakes in data storage as well as entries and maintenance of patient records can occur and can affect the diagnosis and treatment of the patient (Wiederhold, 1980). To illustrate such errors, a case study presented by Hebda and Czar (2005) can be used, and is as follows:

Agnes Gibbons was admitted through the hospital's emergency department with congestive heart failure. During her admission she was asked to verbally acknowledge whether her demographic data were correct. Ms. Gibbons did so. Extensive diagnostics tests were done, including radiology studies. It was later discovered that all of Ms. Gibbons' information had been entered into another client's file (Hebda & Czar, 2005).

As the case study states, Ms. Gibbons participated in the process of her positive identification through the use of informatics. Nevertheless, her health information was placed under the wrong file by the nurse. This type of error occurred as a result of the healthcare provider not having sufficient understanding of the technology in use.

The company should be given the name of the clients that were affected, the corrections that were made, and inquiries about a plan that could prevent the same thing happening again. In this situation, it is important to remember that "although the initial data collection and entry process provides an excellent opportunity to verify data accuracy and completeness, it should not be the only time that is done" (Hebda & Czar, 2005, p. 64). In this situation, we could improve the way we use informatics in nursing by having the nurse ask the client to review the printouts entered in the data to recheck the given information. The lesson would be that it is important to continuously review the data as you are giving care; it was the only way the nurse found the error. By working with other departments in the healthcare field, we are increasing the number of eyes that review information and are therefore giving more people the ability to identify the errors. The nurse who made an error in this case study would need to inform all the hospital departments (starting from her unit manager; it is not the nurse's responsibility to inform all the departments) that were giving the client services. For example, the radiology department, the ER, and laboratory, in case they access the client information and to avoid any complication to the client. Perhaps one of the departments might have caught the mistake and informed her of the error before she even realized it. By increasing human review on the attained information, nurses can reduce the amount of errors and improve patients' care.

Being in the healthcare field not only requires one to know the skills needed, it also includes one to have a critical thinking mind to help give the best care. Now that we know we have a problem, with nursing informatics data verification we can correct it. Agnes Gibbons's error would need to be dealt with immediately. At first, the charge nurse or nurse manager would be notified. He or she should understand the nature of the error in question. This would allow proper filing of an incident form or report as necessary. Proper documentation needs to be done so that the proper authorities can be aware of the error, and the patient should be notified that the hospital is doing everything they can to fix it. The patient should then be reassessed to ensure accuracy of any data entered. Furthermore, the nurse who made an error in this case study would need to inform all the hospital departments (not the nurse's responsibility, the chain of command has been previously described), family, and power of attorney as required by the facility.

The fact remains that all healthcare providers responsible for identifying data errors use critical thinking to prevent, improve, and even correct data errors. These errors should try to be found and then those who make them should be reeducated about the use of the technology in question to prevent repeating of the same error (Hallbach & Sullivan, 2005). Informatics is a great tool to have in the healthcare field to make our job not only more accurate, but also more efficient. We have to keep in mind our responsibility to continue educating ourselves in new technologies and improvement techniques. Human error will always exist because human beings are not perfect, but it is our duty to do no harm intentionally and therefore find solutions to better improve our practice. Regardless of whether errors are made, the most important goal and focus is to provide excellent healthcare service to the patient. If excellent service is being provided, then healthcare providers are doing their jobs and doing them to the best of their ability.

In addition, medical devices are to be routinely evaluated for expiration, accuracy, and proper functionality to ascertain patient safety as Zhang, Johnson, Patel, Paige, and Kubose (2003) correctly concluded in their investigation.

Heuristic evaluation can be used to identify a great proportion of major usability problems in a product in a timely manner with reasonable cost. Human errors in medical device use are largely due to interface design problems that can be potentially addressed through user-centered design, interventions, and other considerations. Since heuristic evaluation can identify usability problems, whose quantity and severity are strongly linked to the frequency of medical errors, heuristic evaluation is a method for indirectly assessing patient safety features in medical devices. Although it is limited in its scope of coverage of the full range of patient safety related features in medical devices, it is a practical tool that should be adopted by medical device manufacturers for the design and modification of medical devices, and by healthcare institutions for the evaluation of medical devices (p. 30, https://doi.org/10.1016/S1532-0464(03)00060-1)

References

American Nurses Association. (2001). *Code of ethics for nurses with interpretive statements* (View Only for Members and Non-Members). Retrieved from https://www.nursingworld.org/practice-policy/nursing-excellence/ethics/code-of-ethics-for-nurses/coe-view-only/

Garrett, R. K., & Danziger, J. N. (2008). Disaffection or expected outcomes: Understanding personal Internet use during work. Disaffection or expected outcomes: Understanding personal Internet use during work. *Journal of Computer-Mediated Communication 13*(4), 937–958.

Halbach J. L., & Sullivan L. L. (2005). Teaching medical students about medical errors and patient safety: Evaluation of a required curriculum. *Academic Medicine, 80*(6), 600–606.

Hebda, T. L., & Czar, P (2005). *Handbook of informatics for nurses and healthcare professionals* (5th ed.). New York, NY: Pearson.

Hebda, T. & Czar, P. (2009). *Handbook of informatics for nurses and healthcare professionals*. Upper Saddle River, NJ: Pearson.

Kolcaba, K. Y. (1994). A theory of holistic comfort for nursing. *Journal of the American Medical Informatics Association, 3*(2):139–148. https://doi.org/10.1111/j.1365-2648.1994.tb01202.x

McDaniel, R. R., Lanham, H. J., & Anderson, R. A. (2009). Implications of complex adaptive systems theory for the design of research on health care organizations. *Health Care Manage Review, 34*(2), 191–199.

Ommaya, A. K., P. F. Cipriano, D. B. Hoyt, K. A. Horvath, P. Tang, H. L. Paz, M. S. DeFrancesco, S. T. Hingle, S. Butler and C. A. Sinsky (2018). Care-Centered Clinical Documentation in the Digital Environment: Solutions to Alleviate Burnout. *National Academy of Medicine Perspectives.* Discussion Paper, National Academy of Medicine, Washington, DC. doi: 10.31478/201801c

Riedy M. K., (2016). Yes, Your Personal Data Is at Risk: Get over It, 19 SMU Science & Technology Law Review. 19,1, p. 3. Available at: https://scholar.smu.edu/scitech/vol19/iss1/2

Schultz, D. (2012). As patient records go digital, theft and hacking problems grow. *Kaiser Health News.* Retrieved from https://khn.org/news/electronic-health-records-theft-hacking/

Singleton, S. (2001) *Encryption and Healthcare Policy Competitive Enterprise Institute: Free market and limited government.* Retrieved from https://cei.org/outreach-regulatory-comments-and-testimony/encryption-and-health-care-policy

Sankar, P., Moran, S., Merz, J. F., & Jones, N. L. (2003). Patient perspectives on medical confidentiality. *Journal of General Internal Medicine, 18*(8), 659–669. Retrieved from http://psycnet.apa.org/record/2003-99937-008

Smith, H. J., Dinev, T., & Xu, H. (2011). Information privacy research: An interdisciplinary review. *MIS Quarterly, 35*(4), 989-1015. Retrieved from https://www.researchgate.net/publication/220260183_Information_Privacy_Research_An_Interdisciplinary_Review

Wiederhold, G. (1980). Databases in healthcare. Stanford Computer Science Department, *CS Report STAN CS80-790*. Retrieved from http://infolab.stanford.edu/pub/gio/1980/CS-TR-80-790.pdf

Zander, P. E. (2008). Ways of knowing in nursing: The historical evolution of a concept. Journal of Theory Construction & Testing, 11(1), 7.

Zhang, J., Johnson, T. R., Patel, V. L., Paige, D. L., & Kubose, T. (2003). Using usability heuristics to evaluate patient safety of medical devices. *Journal of Biomedical Informatics, 36*(1-2), 23-30.

UNIT V

CHAPTER 13

Digital Library and Mobile Computing

CHAPTER HIGHLIGHTS

This chapter discusses the following:

- How surge in information and technology has affected the library and access to digital library is inevitable
- How health datasets have made nurses, nursing students, and faculty stay current in their profession, and more importantly provide evidence-based care (EBP).
- How tablets have offered healthcare professional's portable computers with which they can document patient care information, review labs, and X-ray images and have enabled the users to carry hundreds of books and periodicals with ease

IN THE PAST, scholarly health information was found only in printed journals and libraries. The healthcare consumers were dependent on health providers for all their information and needs. With the advent of Internet in the 1990s, the consumer has access to as much information as the healthcare provider. The libraries continue to be a resource for knowledge and evidence-based practice (EBP). This surge in information and technology has affected the library, and access to digital library is inevitable. The Andrew W. Mellon Foundation report on the Future of the Academic Library Print Collection: A Space for Engagement has reiterated the need for digital libraries as follows:

> Academic and special libraries are in the middle of a shift towards hybrid collections. This shift has led to demands for remote services, which is complicated for collection and management. It is impossible for libraries to meet the demand and anticipated needs of nurses and healthcare institution needed to manage patient care. As students and faculty increasingly expect and need immediate desktop access to abstracts and full text, collection developers are dramatically trading off ownership of print materials to pay for licenses to access electronic services. Libraries have turned to inter-organization arrangements, consortia and licensing to provide access to necessary materials. (p. 2)

Librarians created index guides to assist with information searches for the literature electronically. These index guides are created as bibliographic databases, which can also be searched electronically. Print card catalogues, annual print indexes of periodic literature, have been replaced by bibliographic databases. Electronic databases are flexible and easy to use. One of the advantages of electronic media is that it eliminates the use of paper and makes more information available to the public. Users can access information electronically in the form of citations, abstracts, and full-text journal articles or textbooks. These types of information are available and indexed in the online database.

The digital database is divided into two categories, which includes knowledge-based databases and factual databases. Knowledge-based data relates to publishing literature, and factual data replaced reference books with searchable and up-to-date information available on line. The focus of knowledge databases is health science, law, ethics, history, and government. The number and types of resources are categorized by each database. Library vendors sell electronic databases to libraries, which helps them offer different electronic resources. Each database has its own search interface window, which identifies the vendor. Some of the major databases that produce health science are *EBSCO, Ovid*, and *ProQuest*. These databases are important to nurses, nursing students, and faculty to stay current in their profession and, more importantly, to provide evidence-based care (EBP).

EVIDENCE-BASED PRACTICE STEPS

Some of the major database useful to nurses are *EBSCO, CINAHL, Medline/PubMed, PsycInfo, Ovid, ProQuest,* and *Cochrane*. Some of the databases include only citations, and abstracts, and others contain full-text documents. *EBSCO* has links to the main menu in the search window. The *Ovid* search window provides tutorials specifically for users. It is important to be familiar with the way the vendor handles Boolean terminology such as (and, or, and not) truncation and wildcards with asterisks, (*) and question marks (?). Truncation is used for variations in spelling. Some of the databases may allow users to restrict online searches to peer-reviewed articles in scholarly journals, articles with references and abstracts, research articles, or full-text articles. Journals are scholarly publications that have been peer reviewed. Articles in magazines, newsletters, newspapers should be used as points of information and entertainment and should not be used to support nursing knowledge. Some of the effective literature search strategies to support evidence-based practice (EBP) include the following:

- Questioning practice and recognizing the information needed; it is the first step in the quest for knowledge. Perform an appropriate search for evidence; literature review is very important in developing EBP. Perform a critical analysis of literature review; it is at this point that knowledge is discovered.
- Systematically implementing the research findings and evaluating the result and effectiveness of practice.
- Applying and implementing search findings.

STRATEGIES FOR ONLINE LITERATURE SEARCH

There are many other ways to perform an online search, including using keywords and federated searches, which performs a search on more than one database. Most of the library vendors search windows allows users to select a citation and format and save the search results. The result of the findings can be e-mailed, printed, or exported to a personal reference manager. Personal reference managers are databases that allow users to create a collection of citations. Most library databases have an export feature, which allows the user to download information to a personal reference manager. Some of the products available are Endnote, ProCite, Reference Manager, and Refworks. There are some free online personal managers such as Zotero. It is a powerful resource because it has the ability to hyperlink files and images and also captures screenshots on Web pages. It is compatible with software such as Openoffice.org and Google Docs. One good quality of Zotero is that it can be used online and offline. Apart from importing citations, it is capable of file synchronization, which is a free service that requires registration, login, and password.

INTEGRATION OF NURSING KNOWLEDGE INTO CLINICAL PRACTICE

Evidence-based practice (EBP) findings and nursing knowledge must be integrated into clinical practice to patient outcomes. There are numerous library guides and tutorials that may be found online, and librarian assistants are available to help with developing competency in searching for information. Specific library facilities have guides to search for information, such as medical subject headings (MeSH) and using a vendor search interface and specific databases. Subject headings relate to standardized terms used in referencing or citing a catalog. Each library database uses subject headings to index materials so that the database can be searched. MeSH refers to various forms of controlled vocabulary used to index materials in *PubMed, Medline,* and *Cumulative Index to Nursing and Allied Health Literature* (CINAHL). It is important to understand the difference in search structure.

The libraries are changing and so are the various facets of business and personal use. There is an increase in demand in the use for mobile technology such as tablets computers, e-readers, digital assistants (PDA), and e-books. As a result of this wireless technology, nurses and other healthcare providers are interested in using these devices at the point of need. This increase in demand for mobile technology has sparked competition between the major technology developers and retailers. According to Brosco (2011).

10.1 million tablets and 6 million e-readers were shipped worldwide. The United [States] accounted for three quarters of the worldwide e-readers in 2010. It is also forecasted that shipments of e-readers will increase to 14.7 million (p. 775).

The personal data assistant (PDA) concept was developed in the early 1980s; iPod PDA was introduced by Apple in 2001, and iPod touch and iPhone were released in 2007. It was designed for personal information management. IBM introduced the first smart phone in 1993 with combined features of cellular phones and Dim software.

MOBILE COMPUTING

Today, smartphones are small computers that have multiple software programs. The word "handheld" refers to all handheld mobile devices. The cell phone is a communication device that has a wireless. The word "cell" refers an area of transmission. This communication does not come free and requires a paid subscription. Most of the software have differences and similarities. Mobile computers have a different operating system but are designed to be interoperable. The various hardware include the following:

- Display: This refers to screen display and resolution. Touch screen is one of the features included for data input. The display ranges from 3.5 inches to 9.7 inches.
- Resolution: This plays an important role with regards to image: The higher the resolution, the sharper the image. It is an important component to consider if video usage is considered.
- Battery: All mobile operating systems use batteries. Most mobile computers use rechargeable batteries.
- Memory: There are three types of built-in memory, namely read-only memory (ROM), which requires a small amount of battery usage and stores add-on applications and data files.
- Random access memory (RAM): This is sensitive to battery life and data may be lost if it is completely depleted.
- Built-in flash memory: This is nonvolatile, which means that data will not be lost if the battery is depleted. PDAs and smartphones do not have a hard drive.
- Data entry: Devices such as iPod Touch, iPod, iPhone, and Nook allow for data entry using the touch of a finger on a screen or stylus.
- Synchronization: Most mobile devises are interoperable with personal computers so that all files can coincide with the computers. The palm devices uses hot sync, and Windows mobile devices transfer data between the mobile device and the PC. Apple uses iTunes to transfer data.
- Connectivity: Depending on the type of mobile device, there are several ways of connecting with other devices or the Internet. Some of the features include beaming, Wi-Fi, and cellular phone lines.
- Beaming: This allows for the transmission of information between short ranges within the same operating system. It is used to share files such as contact information, calendar, or documents such as Word or Excel with another device.
- Bluetooth: This allows for connection to other Bluetooth-enabled devices. It can be used to synchronize a mobile device with a PC or printer and also listen to music, podcasts, and other audio media.
- Wi-Fi: It is an industry standard and also a means of mobile device connectivity. It is an acronym for wireless fidelity, which uses a router. Wi-Fi is very popular because it allows multiple users in the family to access printers and the Internet. A "hotspot" is a means of identifying a Wi-Fi-enabled area to use a device. All hotspots are not free; some are encrypted and require an access code or payment for access.

Advantages: Some of the advantages with the use of handheld devices include time saving and time management, patient safety error reduction, ease of looking up references, quality of care, and elimination of pushing drug carts. When updates are available, they can easily be downloaded and saved on a mobile device. PDAs are used in medication administration, which has reduced medication errors. The PDA is wireless and as such facilitates data updates. For example, as soon as a patient is admitted, the patient's name shows on the list for that unit, the pharmacy verifies the meds once they are ordered, and they show up on that list. The use of handheld devices would improve patient care. Most nurses have their own handheld device to provide point of reference information for decision making. Handheld devices are an important asset to nursing research. They are excellent tools for collecting and assessing data. They are assets to nurses in all settings. Nursing students are expected to use handheld devices in the classroom as well as in clinical settings.

Disadvantages: Some of the disadvantages include high cost of PDAs, rapid change in technology, occasional issues with family devices, and short battery life. One of the most important problems to consider with handheld devices is security. Data security is always an issue with small wireless devices. They must be encrypted using a password or biometrics.

In conclusion, advanced technologies, handheld computers, are an important tool for nurses to gather information from the palm of their hands. Users can read books, store references, and use them in clinical practice. It is an added value to nurses in all settings. This new wave of technology will help in decision making, improve accuracy of documentation, and decrease the amount of time spent between the delivery of care and documentation through electronic media.

> As tablets and e-reader increase in popularity, businesses and professionals in all fields will need to look at the service they offer. Tablets [in] healthcare offer the professionals['] portable computers with which they can document patient care information, review labs, and x-ray images. It allows the users to carry hundreds of books and periodicals with ease. The key will be how to trim down the number of devices to carry. Although security will always be a major concern, new technologies will be developed to combat these problems. (Brusco, 2011, p. 775)
>
> Libraries today are striving to meet the demands of their customers. Many have integrated new technology trends to such as e-books, [and] social media sites such as Facebook, Foursquare, Twitter [are] creating mobile interfaces to their catalogs and databases to bring electronic resources and library information to mobile device. (Avery, 2011)

The PDA will continue to be used in the improvement of patient care and education in the classroom, and popularity will also continue to grow and evolve through many years to come.

References

Andrew W. Mellon Foundation report on the Future of the Academic Library Print Collection: A Space for Engagement (2018), p1–50. Retrieved from https://lib.asu.edu/sites/default/files/marketing/ASU%20Whitepaper%20-%20Which%20Books.pdf

Brusco, J. M., (2011). Tablet and e-reader technology in health care and education. *AORN Journal, 83*(6), 775–781. Retrieved from https://aornjournal.onlinelibrary.wiley.com/doi/abs/10.1016/j.aorn.2011.04.001

Covi, L. M., & Cragin, M. H. (2003). Reconfiguring control in library collection development: A conceptual framework for assessing the shift toward electronic collections. *Journal of the American Society for Information Science and Technology, 55*(4), 312–325.

CHAPTER 14

E-Learning, Teaching, and Author's Related Projects

CHAPTER HIGHLIGHTS

This chapter discusses the following:

- Why emphasis on exploring alternate methods of delivery and credentialing to accommodate a rapidly increasing student population and the diversity of their needs is the new paradigm
- How e-learning not only introduced a sharp growth in the size of distance learning business, but also has become an accepted means of acquiring knowledge in our globalized world
- How wider application of knowledge-based and skills-based learning are supported through the many-to-many online teaching methods
- The advantages and disadvantages of online teaching/learning and the factors that contribute to the success of the online learner

IN THEIR EXECUTIVE summary Johnson and colleagues reminded us of the future of education through the following questions:

> What is on the five-year horizon for higher education institutions? Which trends and technology developments will drive educational change? What are the challenges that we consider as solvable or difficult to overcome, and how can we strategize effective solutions? These questions and similar inquiries regarding technology adoption and educational change steered collaborative research and discussions in education today" of a body of 58 experts to produce the NMC Horizon Report: 2016 Higher Education Edition, in partnership with the EDUCAUSE Learning Initiative (Johnson, Adams Becker, Cummins, Estrada, Freeman, and Hall (2016, p. 1).

E-TEACHING/LEARNING

As nurse educators are continuously challenged to stay current in today's complex healthcare, the environment continues to rapidly expand in the field of nursing informatics.

Nurse educators' expectations range from electronic health records, social media, consumer informatics, mobile-health, smart phones, and other applications to prepare students for a data, information, and technology intensive healthcare environment. In addition, there are high expectations from current students who have grown up in the information age and already possess advanced computer skills. Also, compounding these challenges is the information technology that is enabling tools to link data, information, knowledge and wisdom and is facilitating problem solving and decision making. (University of Minnesota, School of Nursing, 2016)

All over the world, universities and colleges have been redesigning their learning spaces to accommodate the new pedagogies and active learning models described across a number of topics in this report. Traditional classroom setups that position rows of seats in front of a podium are being remodeled to facilitate deeper learning experiences and interactions. (Johnson et al., 2016, p. 7)

However, incorporating information technology in ways that educate students on these important concepts remain a challenge for many educators, and this has been my call and strength as a nurse informatics specialist (NIS).

The Innovation Policy Platform (IPP) asserts that universities should bolster entrepreneurship courses to attract and accommodate more students, while nurturing faculty that can meet high-quality teaching standards. Educators in these programs must understand the complex pedagogies that support more 9 interactive learning; universities should even encourage faculty and staff to hone their own entrepreneurial skills through professional development and opportunities to participate in startups. The IPP recommends that training policies move beyond business development and management to emphasize the challenges of enterprise growth, risk-taking, and building strategic alliances. (p. 8–9)

In one of the author's published articles, Okunji & Hill, 2014 tested a model for a hybrid (60%) leadership online course. The overall assessment showed that the interrelationship between faculty (receptivity to academic concerns, dedication to quality learning experience) and students (career preparation, personal growth, job enhancements) resulted into student satisfaction (academic performance and educational experience).

Faculty dedication and students' satisfaction of the

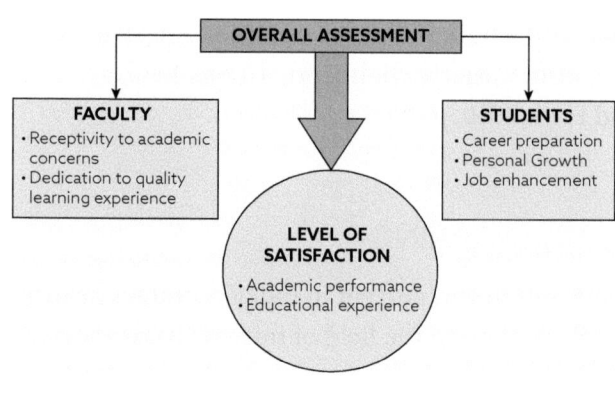

FIGURE 14.1

Source: Okunji P. O., Hill, M (2013). Undergraduate Online Program Development, Implementation and Evaluation: A Pilot Study. *Canadian Journal of Nursing Informatics*, Summer/Fall 2013, 8 (3 & 4), 1-9. URL http://cjni.net/journal/?tag=priscilla-okunji

program were highly significant when compared with overall quality of the program with 99.6% of the predictors explained in the study. Hence, this study has demonstrated that faculty dedication and student satisfaction are critical variables when planning the integration of an online teaching and learning in any institution of higher learning. (Okunji & Hill, 2014, p. 1, 5–6)

Therefore, effective teaching focuses on conveying accurate information and using innovative communications techniques for students' satisfactory outcome. I am the coordinator of all the 11 online RN-BSN core courses (Role Transition, Health Assessment, Nursing Issues, Nursing Concepts, Nursing Informatics and Technology, Nursing Ethics, Nursing Research, Nursing Policy, Nursing Leadership, Community/Mental Health Nursing and Death and Dying). Out of these courses, I currently teach Role Transition, in both hybrid (60% online and 40% face to face) and online (100%) settings, Nursing Informatics and Technology, and online leadership courses. The Nursing Informatics (NI) course is my primary course, which serves as the foundation and conveys the principles of nurses as knowledge workers because NI is based on the theoretical framework that data (biometrics that nurses collect) are critical when interpreted into information and information, when compared, gives us the knowledge and knowledge experience that equates to wisdom, which enables healthcare providers to make informed decisions for patients' well-being. Information cannot become knowledge by itself, except with critical thinking and the cognitive, intellectual, and analytical ability of the nurse that transforms data collected into useful knowledge in EHR.

In the last few years, e-learning has not only introduced a sharp growth in the size of distance learning business, but also has become an accepted means of acquiring knowledge in our globalized world. The rapid advancement in computer technology, the availability of plethora online teaching methods, and the easy accessibility of the Internet have made learning more inclusive and easier. In other words, unlike some decades ago, when people could blame their lack of knowledge and/or inability to achieve their academic goals on work/family-related responsibilities, the difficulties created by distances, and to some extent on economic constraints, with online leaning students are able to manage their time better to accommodate other personal, family, and worked-related needs. It is even truer since e-learning has become a major part of the current educational system. Consequently, it is plausible to say that e-learning has come about because of the demands of learners, as well as the growth and fast expansion of computer technology.

Nonetheless, the advantages of online learning have not come on a platter of gold; as a result, e-learning has some loopholes. Students who are not self-disciplined or motivated, and/or students with poor knowledge of computers, find e-learning very frustrating and either they end up not finishing their course or do very poorly at the end of the program. With all this in mind, this paper will discuss the general concepts relating to educational informatics by paying particular attention to Bloom's taxonomy of learning. It will also examine the effective way to this learning by comparing computerized quizzing and survey features with those of printed versions and by depicting how online databases of teaching/learning resources such as the MERLOT project benefit learners.

The paper will not be limited on these issues only, but will discuss some of the strengths and weaknesses of e-learning, interpret the factors affecting distance education outcomes, and examine the role of the student in distance education. Before the conclusion this paper, I will identify and explain three essential characteristics that, if properly followed, would contribute immensely to the success of students who take course(s) online. Finally, I will conclude by arguing that the problems and the difficulties that are associated with e-leaning can be controlled by students and administrators being diligent.

Different online teaching methods contribute to learning basing on Bloom's taxonomy of learning. Bloom's taxonomy of learning uses three main categories: knowledge, skills, and effective tools (Wyatt & White, 2007). Online teaching methods support the Bloom taxonomy of learning through the different techniques they apply. Online teaching methods are also categorized in terms of how knowledge is retrieved. Initially, the retrieval of information is individual based, where only one student accomplishes the learning task without communicating with other students (Stavredes, 2011). This level of learning would still be very much theoretical as the student gains knowledge and theories and comprehends such data according to knowledge-based goals. Sources for these knowledge-based goals include the use of online databases, online journals, online applications, and software libraries (Stavredes, 2011). Improvements in knowledge-based goals are also observed through online teaching methods such as learning contracts, apprenticeships, internships, and correspondence studies (Stavredes, 2011).

ONLINE STUDENTS' INTERACTION

Interaction with other students and with society covers skill-based and effective goals. This can be seen in the online teaching methods that have a wider interaction with the outside world. This includes lectures, symposiums, and skits (Buzzetto-More, 2011). The student is gradually using sensory cues to guide user's actions. He or she is also becoming familiar with tools in completing or performing tasks. Confidence in carrying out tasks is also improved through these online teaching methods. New tasks and goals are also established for the learner through lectures and symposiums (Buzzetto-More, 2011). The Bb discussion forum for each module is in the form of topic post, comment and critique (PC^2). The discussion board is an innovation that not only allows for student-to-faculty interactions, but also for students to students deep thinking, especially for the online students, as online interaction is a critical variable in distance learning. PC^2 guides the student to read the initial instructor's post and students respond without reading other students' comments. A time lag is then given for students to read other students' comments and critique on others' responses and comments. Essentially, PC^2 effectively motivates students to think critically. The virtual classroom is another forum for students to voice their intellectual abilities. The author saw the opportunity as a teaching and learning with technology (TLT) institutional committee member and one of the early adopters to pilot the Bb collaboration and Tegrity interactive tools that the University is currently using for teaching and learning.

THE INFORMATICS TEACHING TOOLS

Blackboard Tegrity

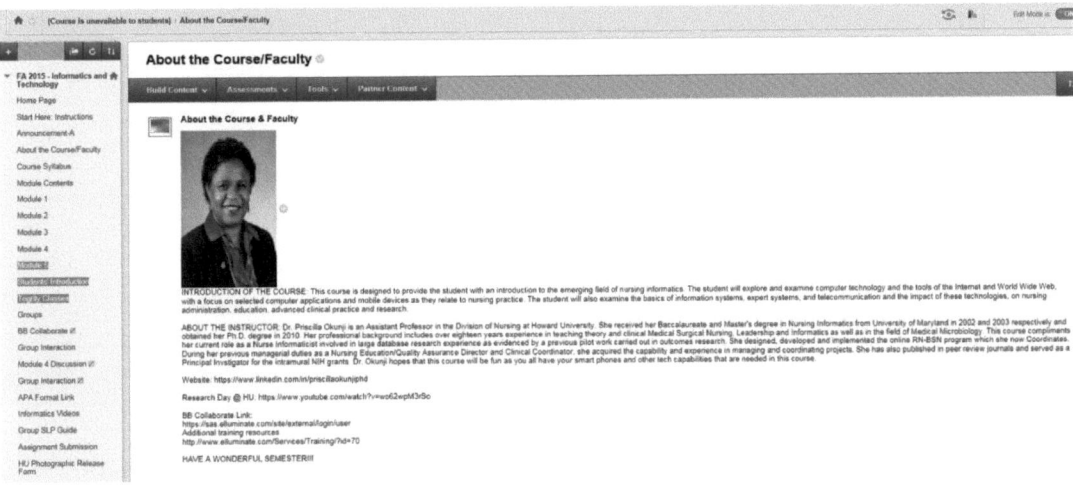

FIGURE 14.2

My Blackboard Informatics Course Webpage Display

A wider application of knowledge-based and skills-based learning is supported through the many-to-many online teaching methods. Such many-to-many methods include tegrity, simulations, wikis, discussion groups, jeopardy, forums, and project groups (Stavredes, 2011). Computer conferencing tools and software such as Blackboard Collaborate, are the primary tools used in the many-to-many approach. Distribution lists for e-mails can also be utilized to maximize the learning process. These computer-mediated learning tools help ensure that the knowledge-based, skills-based, and effective elements of learning are served and stimulated for the learner.

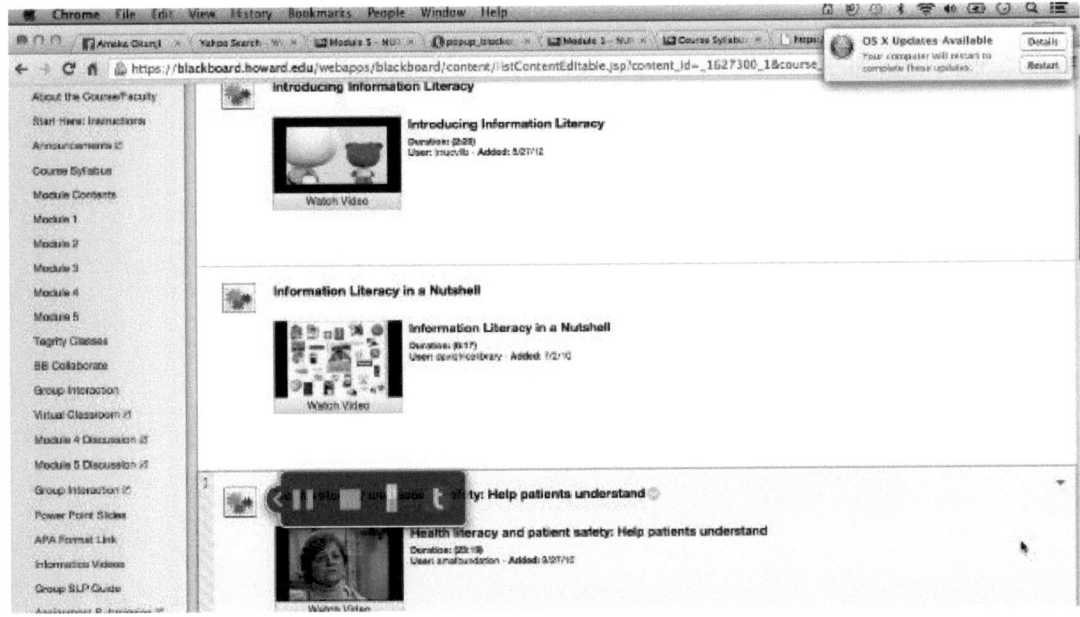

FIGURE 14.3

SimChart (Simulated EHR for Clinical Courses)

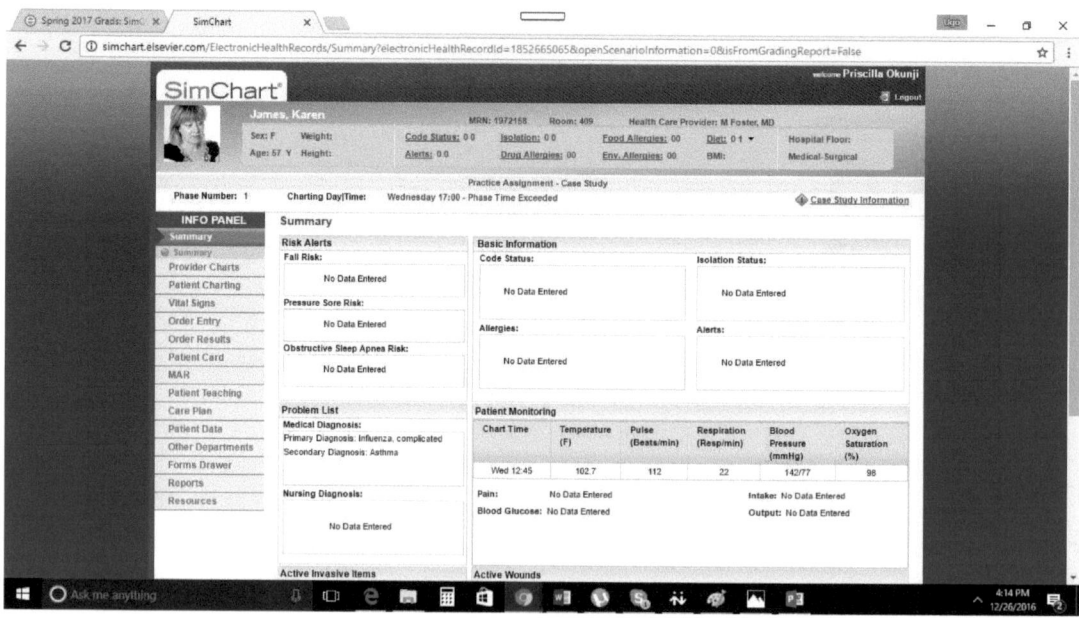

FIGURE 14.4 Simulation station: Courtesy of Urban Hospital Simulation Center

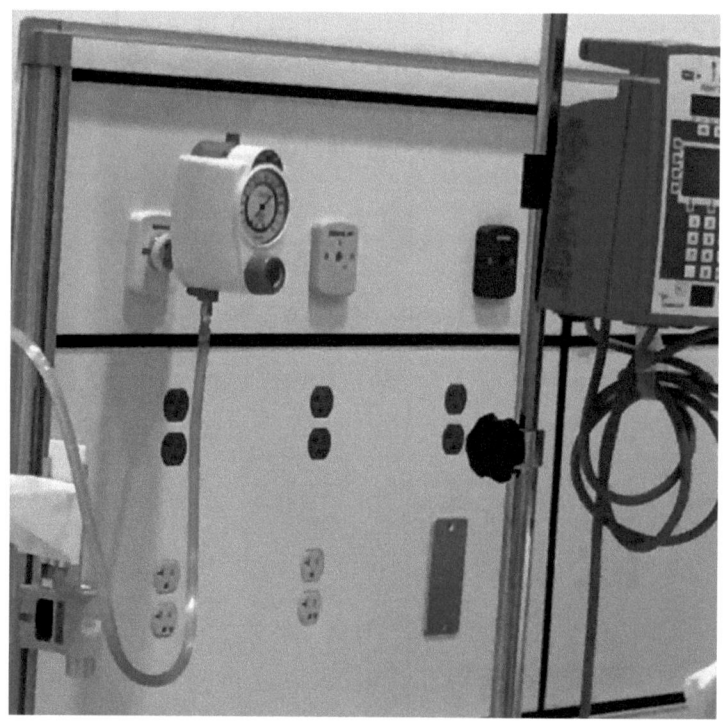

FIGURE 14.5

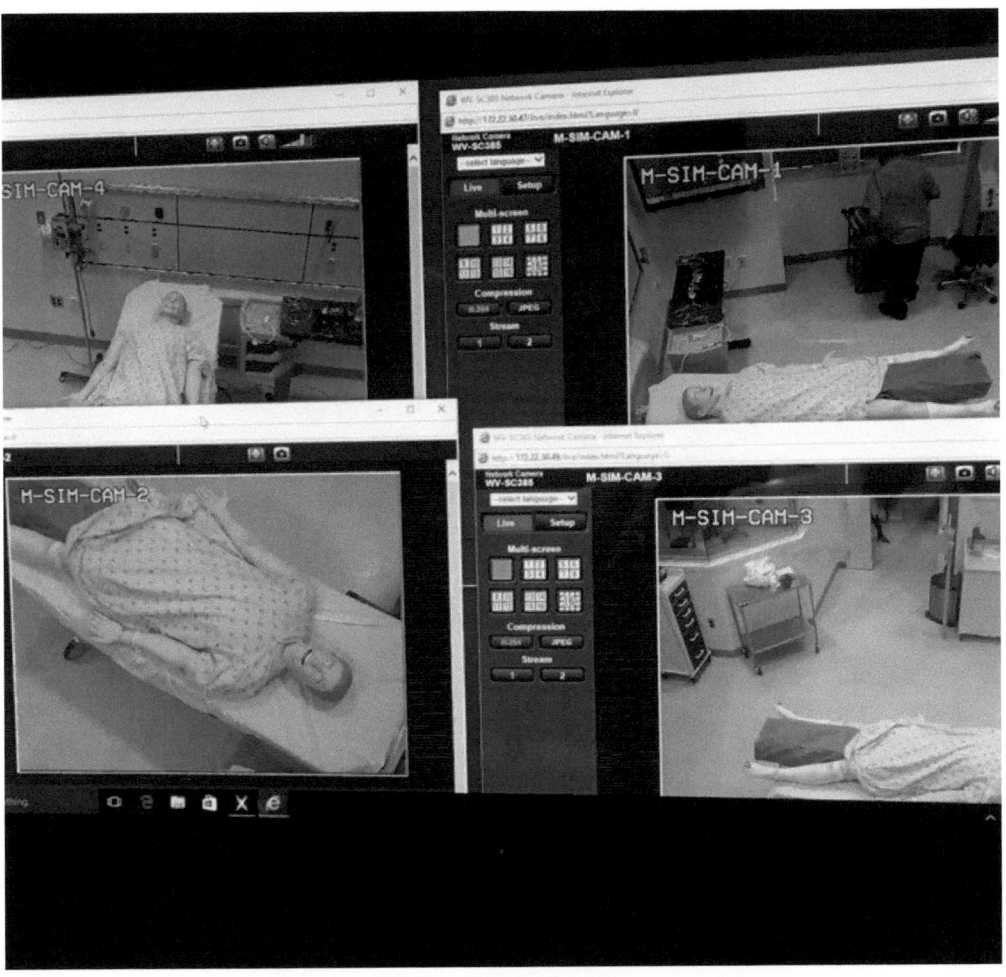

FIGURE 14.6   A Sim-man displayed with a wedge for hip replacement post-op care

Courtesy of Howard University Simulation Center

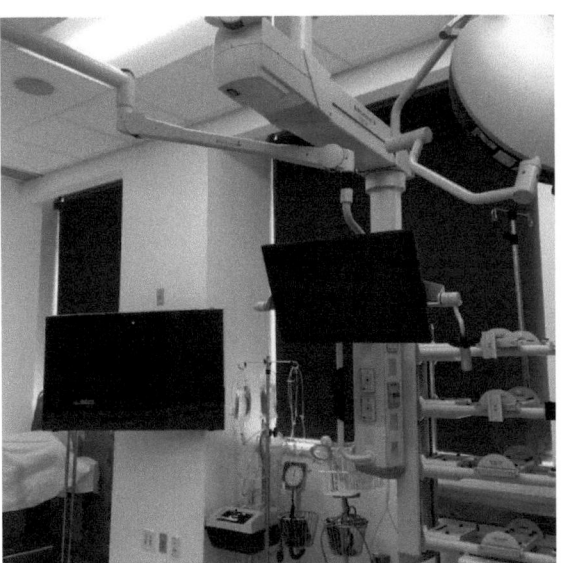

FIGURE 14.7   Simulation scene: Courtesy of Howard University

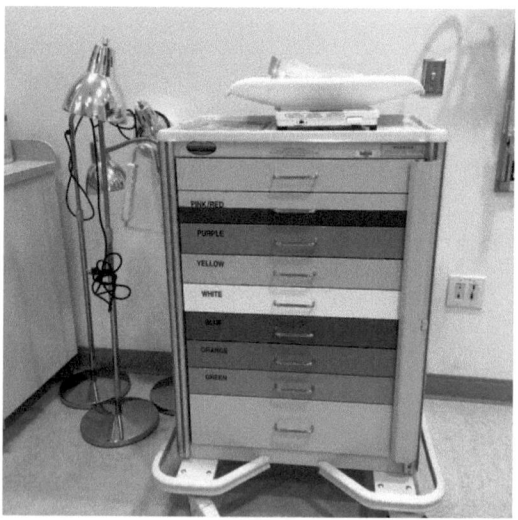

FIGURE 14.8   Unit color coded crash cart simulated

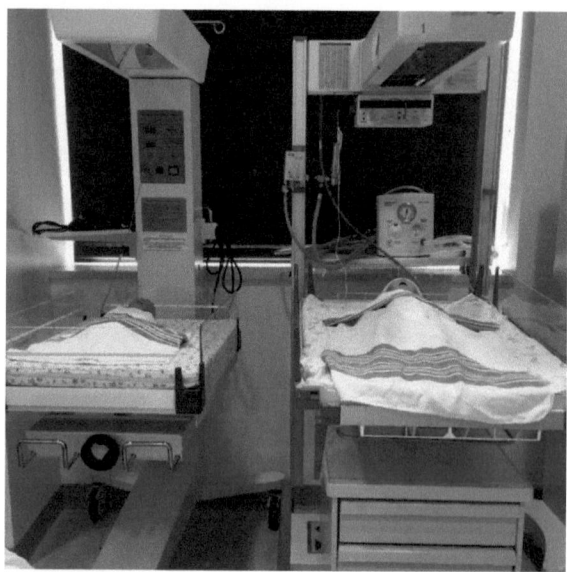

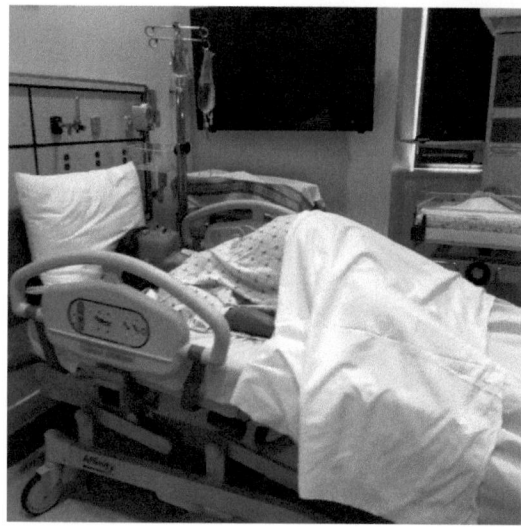
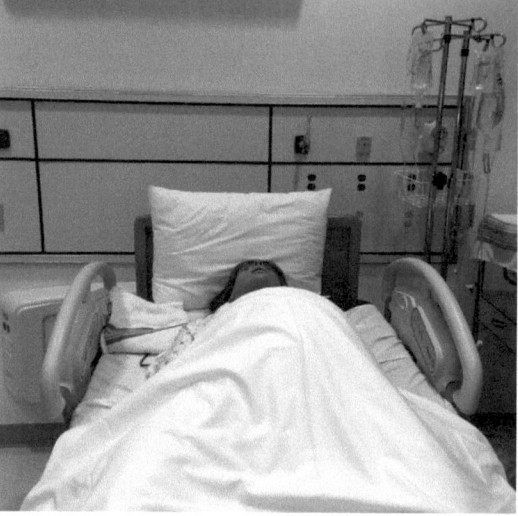

FIGURE 14.9   Mother-baby simulated

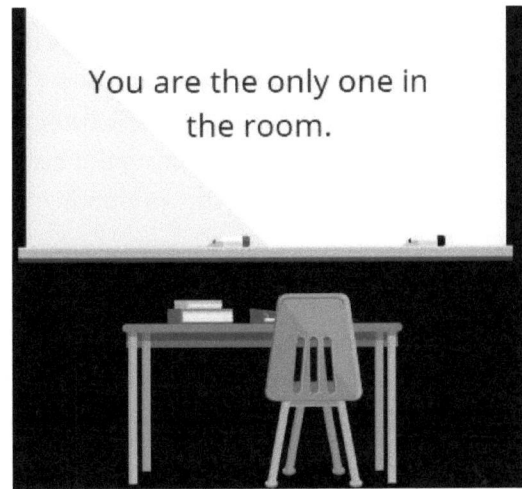

FIGURE 14.10 Bb Collaborate pic

Bb Discussion Board

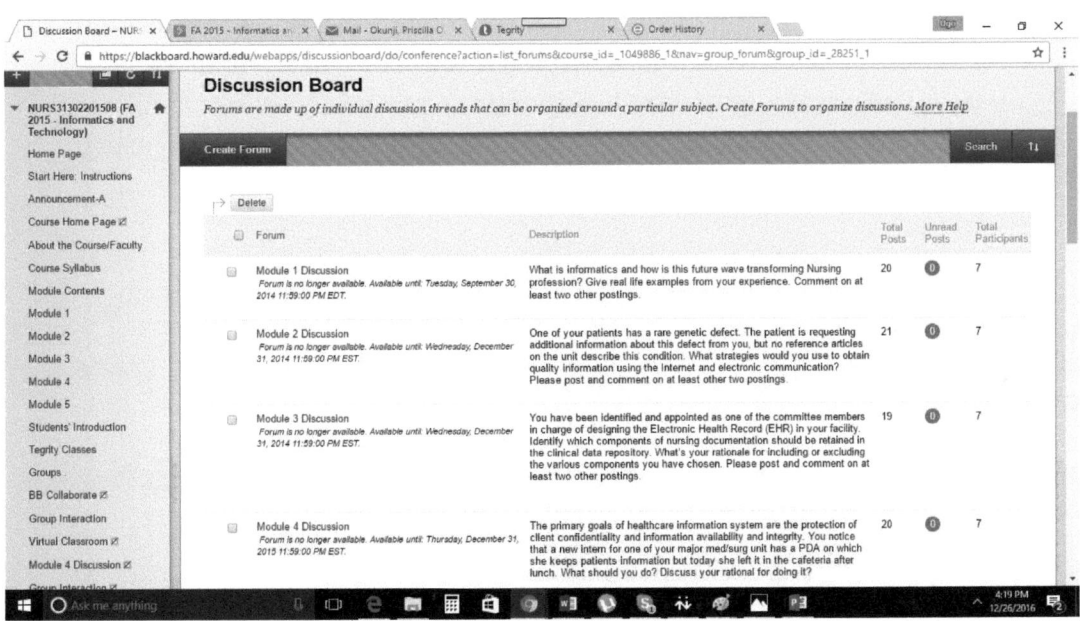

FIGURE 14.11

COMPUTERIZED QUIZZING/TESTING

Computerized quizzing or online surveys differ significantly from print-version quizzes. For computerized surveys, questions can be written with complete and specific descriptions of the questions indicated (Fidelman, 2007). This sometimes is not possible with printed surveys because of space constraints. However, this may not always be true especially in instances when the question is already familiar to respondents. In these instances, no explanation for the questions is indicated in the online quiz. Online surveys also have the ability to include images as well as other formats; audio and video may also accompany the survey (Noyes & Garland, 2008). These elements can then be used by the researchers to highlight aspects of the question which may not be familiar to the respondent.

The author has published an article on the technology integration in undergraduate traditional nursing programs. This article describes a pilot study conducted to survey senior nursing students' responses to online testing preference and the efficiency of the Blackboard system to offer such testing.

> Preparation for online testing was done in phases starting with the planning for the testing space and computer availability. This was followed by selection and uploading of appropriate questions on the course Blackboard® site for student access. The questions were then exported to the testing port of the course web page with certain embedded restrictions. Finally, the survey was developed with seventeen items based on a review of the literature and [was] implemented. Data analysis was performed on student responses on the survey, and results indicated moderate to high support for online testing. The survey analysis indicated that more than half of the students preferred online exams over traditional testing, indicating likability and convenience over traditional scantron paper exams. Most students showed a preference for online testing and recommended that test results be available for immediate review. One advantage to introducing online testing was to foster familiarity with computerized testing as preparation for the NCLEX-RN® licensure exam. (Okunji & Hill, 2014, p. 1)

EXAM SOFT COMPUTERIZED TESTING

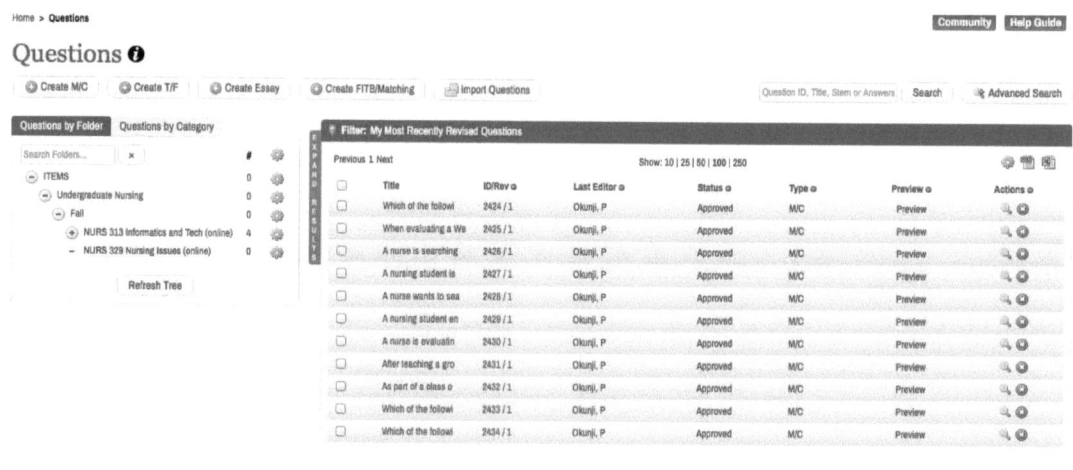

FIGURE 14.12

Online or computerized surveys also have the ability to draw and sustain the attention of the respondent in ways that cannot be made possible through printed surveys or quizzes. Audio-visual features and similar features can capture the readers' attention long enough to complete the survey and ensure high response rates for the survey or quiz (Boyer, Olson, & Jackson, 2001). Merely scrolling and clicking the mouse can accomplish the task of answering the survey, thereby also ensuring high response rates for the questionnaire.

Despite the favorable qualities of these online quizzes or surveys, there are also disadvantages observed in using these quizzes. One glaring issue is the fact that not all individuals are comfortable with computer use (Pflieger, 2008). The older generation certainly is not adept and comfortable with the use of computers. Issues relating to data quality have also been raised. This disparity may be attributed to the presentation, layout, and the biased nature of data collection. The bias comes from the limited monitoring of respondents, which cannot be secured for online respondents (Boyer et al., 2001). Computer issues including lost electronic mail addresses, computer viruses, and technical issues can also compromise the administration and the taking of online quizzes or surveys. So far, this paper has narrated online teaching methods and the difference between online quizzing and printed quizzing, but how does the online database affect students?

The most significant benefit for the centralized online database in learning and teaching relates mostly to its multi-functionality (Liu, 2008). It allows a comprehensive search possibility for students. It also includes a database that is transparent and continuously updated by the online administrator. An overview of the current studies carried out at various locations and areas of study are also indicated in the online databases (Liu, 2008). The subject of these topics can easily be seen, including an overview of the issues proposed as well as recommendations for the practice, for education, and for research. Facts and figures could easily be generated from online databases, by students to understand trends, as well as to understand phenomena.

Through the online databases of teaching and learning, collaborations between the different investigators and universities can be established, allowing the easy creation of daily activities. Actions and recommendations can also be automated by such databases, thereby allowing for the monitoring of these actions, in line with the results of research. Having examined the e-learning methods, the difference of the computerized quiz from printed version and how the online database affects the learner, at this point, this paper will identify and discuss the strengths and the weaknesses of e-learning methods.

E-LEARNING STRENGTHS AND WEAKNESSES

There are various strengths and weaknesses for e-learning. In general, it is beneficial because it can flexibly be scheduled, and it can be managed based on work, family, and social obligations (Muilenberg & Burge, 2005). Travel time is also decreased with e-learning as students are not required to travel to and from campus. Students are also able to consider choices relating to learning tools, which would meet their needs, their knowledge, and their interest. Students are also able to study and carry out their school activities anywhere as long as they can access a computer and have an Internet connection. The pace of the learning is also based on the student, not the teacher (Muilenberg & Burge, 2005). The students can also easily involve themselves in bulletin board–threaded discussions, even without being in school. Through e-learning methods, teachers and instructors can easily connect and interact with each other. The communication process is faster and easier to carry out. Various teaching styles that support learning can also be made possible with

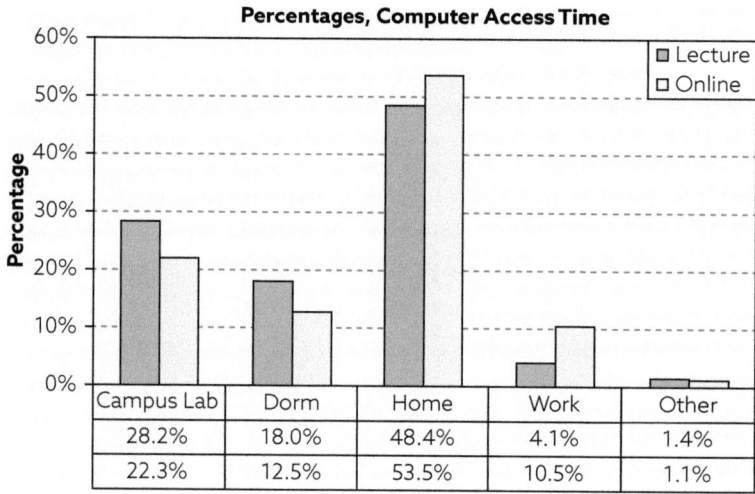

FIGURE 14.13

e-learning (Mbarek & Zaddem, 2013). The skills of students with computers are also enhanced.

Accessibility of computers and Internet technology has been emphasized as a crucial part of online e-learning. As demonstrated in the figure that follows, most students are likely to secure access to the Internet at home or at work, with lecture students using school access for their Internet school work.

These benefits notwithstanding, e-learning also has its weaknesses. Learners who are not highly motivated or who have bad study habits or no discipline will likely fall behind in their school requirements. Some students may also not thrive well without traditional classroom settings, and as a result may be confused in their school activities and requirements (Mbarek & Zaddem, 2013). These students may also feel disconnected from their teacher and classmates due to limited personal interaction with them. Some students may also have simple practical considerations in e-learning with slow or no Internet connection or with a slow computer or no computer. For those with beginner-level computer skills, some students may also fall behind in their lessons (Buzzetto-More, 2007). Finally, the hands-on approach to learning cannot be achieved in the computerized e-learning setup. As such, the quality of learning is diminished. To ensure that the quality of learning is not diminished because one chooses e-learning as a method of acquiring knowledge, this paper will now examine the factors that either facilitate or jeopardize distance educational outcomes.

Factors affecting distance education outcomes are attributed to different factors that relate to students and universities. Distance education learning has slowly expanded in the past few years. As can be seen in the diagram that follows, its coverage and usage has expanded with each academic year. These trends will likely be sustained for many more years to come. Hence, the importance of securing computer accessibility and skills is as important as the learning process itself.

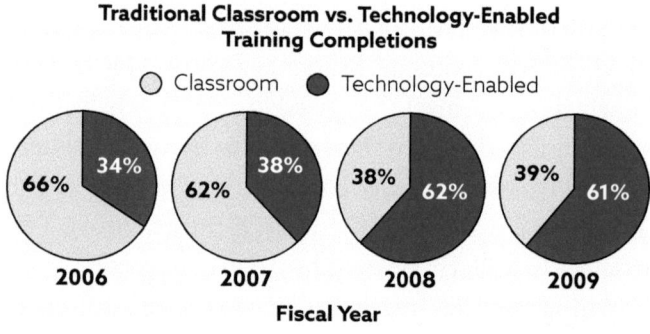

FIGURE 14.14

Computer self-efficacy is a factor that can impact the efficacy of distance education outcomes (Mbarek & Zaddem, 2013). Self-efficacy impacts on the behavior of individuals in terms of execution of actions. In effect, self-efficacy refers to an individual's belief about his or her ability to use resources to accomplish a task. Where a student is not self-efficient in his or her computer use, he or she would not be able to accomplish academic demands and school tasks that are essential to secure academic goals. The students and his or her self-perceived usefulness can also affect the outcomes for distance education learning.

The perceptions on ease of use help indicate and predict the actual intention as well as usage interactions on business areas. Under these conditions, the perceived ease of use refers to the extent by which a learner believes the use of specific system to be free of physical or mental effort (Davis, 2004). Within the online setting, technical support indicates a significant impact on the perceived ease of use of the learning resources (Ngai, Poon, & Chan, 2007). The e-learning process also ensures a useful and interactive interaction between trainees and virtual instructors (Zhang & Zhou, 2003). As such, it helps support the perceived ease of the learning material. Where the distance education facilities provide a structural support for instruction, learning efficacy can be improved.

In some cases, the virtual training setting must manage the communication between the trainees who are physically separated from each other. Through these tools, the perceived ease of use can indicate ease in learning and ease of interaction and eventually can improve future job performance. From what has been argued so far, it is obvious that e-learning has enabled more people to accomplish their educational goals better than traditional classroom methods. However, the success of the e-learning is not only dependent on the availability of computers, Internet connections, e-learning teachers, and administrations. Rather, much of its success is dependent on students' willingness to play their role and abide by the demands and the challenges of e-learning method of learning.

WHAT FACTORS CONTRIBUTE TO THE SUCCESS OF THE ONLINE LEARNER?

The role of the learner in distance education is mostly to learn. This challenging objective calls for motivation, discipline, and planning, as well as the analysis and use of the knowledge being transferred. The challenge for students is to manage various aspects of their life, which often impact each other significantly (Willis, 2003). The student's role is also to become and stay responsible for him- or herself. A significant level of motivation is needed to manage distance courses. In general, there is no daily interaction with students and teachers, and the temptation to stray is strong under these conditions. The student must also know his or her own strength, desire, skill, and needs. He or she must understand his or her goals as well as objectives to ensure direction in his or her activities (Willis, 2003). Students must also do their best to sustain and even increase their self-esteem.

Students must not be afraid and must instead be confident in their ability to manage their studies. Students must also do their best to relate with others to allow for group problem solving. Such problem-solving activities can be secured through group meetings or through computer conferencing (Willis, 2003). It is also important for these students to clarify what they are learning. They therefore have to reflect on what they have learned. They need to assess their existing learning standards on their own and how these can be changed by new data. As such, students are able to understand the need to review their knowledge and its accuracy. Their role therefore also relates to redefining legitimate knowledge. The next paragraph will explain the e-learning essential characteristics that differentiate it from classroom methods.

In reviewing the qualities of learners taking courses online, there are significant essential elements that are associated with successful online learning. One of these essential elements and qualities that a student who uses e-learning as a method of learning must have is a robust motivation to learn (Hoffman, 2003). The student must be invested in the learning process. He or she must be able to do the school work, even with minimal supervision from the teacher. Being a bad student under these conditions would lead to students not doing their school work and falling behind the expected learning outcomes at each stage of the learning process.

Online learners must also be functionally adept in the use of computers. The bulk of the work for distance education requires computer knowledge and moderate computer skills. This would include knowledge in the use of Microsoft Office applications, including Microsoft Word, Microsoft Excel, and Powerpoint, as well as the use of electronic mail, the use of the Internet, and other computer applications. With limited knowledge and skill in these applications, students will fall significantly behind in their school work, most likely causing them to fail their courses (Hoffman, 2003).

However, to ensure the success of distance education, it is also important for students to participate in student forums and bulletin discussion boards. These forums and boards can help them in their learning process. These forums and boards often include students and teachers in their threads (Hoffman, 2003). Teachers can facilitate the discussions and answer student questions and concerns. Students can also help those who may be struggling with their learning. These forums and boards also ensure that students are being steered in the right direction for learning. Online learning, teaching, and development can only have value to the learners if well planned, developed, implemented, and evaluated as needed. The author of this book has published articles related to online development and students testing experience: (1) Okunji and Hill (2013), and (2) Okunji and Hill (2014).

In conclusion, based on the discussion, healthcare is becoming personalized. mHealth could offer personal toolkits for critically needed predictive, participatory, and preventative care. It is apparent that e-learning has become a welcome and necessary addition to learning and academic processes. E-learning has various strengths and weaknesses, and in the current context of widespread computer use, it has also become the more convenient and cost-effective learning tool. The visceral feel of the classroom face-to-face interaction has become superfluous in the context of e-learning. Issues in e-learning relate to problems that would likely be resolved as more developments in computer use are introduced. Under these conditions, the learning process has evolved based on the current conditions of technology. In the end, such developments are current and are very much supportive of academia and the discovery of more information.

References

Boyer, K. K., Olson, J. R., & Jackson, E. C. (2001). Electronic surveys: Advantages and disadvantages over traditional print surveys. *Decision Line, 32*(4), 4–7.

Buzzetto-More, N. (Ed.). (2007). *Principles of effective online teaching*. Santa Rosa, CA: Informing Science Press.

Davis, F. (2004). Perceived usefulness, perceived ease of use, and user acceptance of information technology. *MIS Quarterly, 13*(3), 319–340.

Fidelman, C. (2007). *Course evaluation surveys: In-class paper surveys versus voluntary online surveys.* New York, NY: ProQuest.

Hoffman, R., (2003). *Distance-learning strategies in campus-based translator education*. Germany: GRIN Verlag.

Johnson, L., Adams Becker, S., Cummings, M., Estrada, V., Freeman, A., & Hall, V. (2016). *NMC horizon report: 2016 higher education edition*. Austin, TX: New Media Consortium.

Liu, Z. (2008). *Paper to digital: Documents in the information age*. New York, NY: ABC-CLIO.

Mbarek, R., & Zaddem, F. (2013). The examination of factors affecting e-learning effectiveness. *International Journal of Innovation and Applied Studies, 2*(4), 423–435.

Muilenburg, L. Y., & Berge, Z. L. (2005). Student barriers to online learning: A factor analytic study. *Distance education, 26*(1), 29–48.

Ngai, E. W. T., Poon, J. K. L., & Chan, Y. H. C. (2007). Empirical examination of adoption of WebCT using TAM. *Computers and Education, 48*, 250–267.

Noyes, J. M., & Garland, K. J. (2008). Computer vs. paper-based tasks: Are they equivalent? *Ergonomics, 51*(9), 1352–1375.

Okunji P. O., Hill, M. (2014). Technology Integration in Undergraduate Traditional Nursing Programs: Students Online Testing Experience. *Canadian Journal of Nursing Informatics,* June 20, 9 (1 & 2), 1–8. URL: http://cjni.net/journal/?tag=priscilla-o-okunji

Okunji P. O., Hill, M. (2013). Undergraduate Online Program Development, Implementation and Evaluation: A Pilot Study. *Canadian Journal of Nursing Informatics,* Summer/Fall 2013, 8 (3 & 4), 1–9. URL http://cjni.net/journal/?tag=priscilla-okunji

Pflieger, M. (2008). *An investigation of censorship of printed and online student publications by high school administrators*. New York, NY: ProQuest.

Stavredes, T. (2011). *Effective online teaching: Foundations and strategies for student success.* Hoboken, NJ: Wiley.

University of Minnesota, School of Nursing. (2016). *National nursing informatics deep dive program.* Retrieved from https://www.nursing.umn.edu/outreach/professional-development/national-nursing-informatics-deep-dive-program, 2016

Willis, B. D. (Ed.). (2003). *Distance education: Strategies and tools*. Englewood Cliffs, NJ: Educational Technology Publishing.

Wyatt, R., & White, E. (2007). *Making your first year a success: A classroom survival guide for middle and high school teachers*. Thousand Oaks, CA: Corwin Press.

Zhang, D. & Zhou, L. (2003). Enhancing e-learning with interactive multimedia. *Information Resources Management Journal, 16*(4), 1–14.

Figure Credits

Fig. 14.2: Copyright © by Blackboard Inc.
Fig. 14.3: Copyright © by Blackboard Inc.
Fig. 14.4: Copyright © by Elsevier Inc.
Fig. 14.10: Copyright © by Blackboard Inc.
Fig. 14.11: Copyright © by Blackboard Inc.
Fig. 14.12: Copyright © by ExamSoft.
Fig. 14.13: Copyright © 2005 by John Dutton and Marilyn Dutton.

CHAPTER 15

Faculty Development via Author's Selected Scholarly E-Learning Articles

Undergraduate Online Program Development, Implementation and Evaluation: A Pilot Study

By Priscilla O. Okunji, Ph.D., RN-BC, INS; & Mary H. Hill, DSN., RN,
Howard University, School of Nursing and Allied Health, Washington DC Division of Nursing

ABSTRACT

THIS ARTICLE PRESENTS an exploration of the development, evaluation and program review of a newly implemented online undergraduateRN (Registered Nurses) to BSN (Bachelor of Science in Nursing) degree program. This process included the incorporation of informatics into the new curriculum, development of a program brochure and flyers for student recruitment, course module design, development of the synchronized and a-synchronized learning platform, student and faculty need assessment and orientation tools as well as development of data sets and analysis for the program evaluation. A one year academic review indicated that the overall assessment of the program was confirmed and predicted by the faculty characteristics, students' professional/personal gain and level of satisfaction. Faculty dedication and students satisfaction of the program were highly significant when compared with overall quality of the program with 99.6% of the predictors explained in this study. Hence, this study has demonstrated that faculty dedication and student satisfaction are critical variables when planning the integration of online teaching and learning in any institution of higher learning.

Keywords: Online, Undergraduate, Informatics, Integration, Curriculum, nursing education, program review, curriculum development

INTRODUCTION

Today, many educators and policy makers view online education as the wave of the future. Students are eligible to apply for financial aid (a change in recent years), online delivery provides schedule flexibility, cost effectiveness and does not require students to relocate to a new place to attend classes or forgo full time employment. This mode of learning favors international students and military personnel working overseas. Taking online classes

Priscilla O. Okunji and Mary H. Hill, "Undergraduate Online Program Development, Implementation and Evaluation: A Pilot Study," *Canadian Journal of Nursing Informatics*, vol. 8, no. 3 & 4. Copyright © 2013 by Canadian Journal of Nursing Informatics. Reprinted with permission.

allows students to not only remain in their current positions in their respective countries while attending classes but could save space, time and money for both students and educational institutions. These benefits can provide more time for faculty scholarly activities and added value to the bottom line of any institution and group of students. This approach also supports the accumulation of documents, transcripts, virtual classroom activity, wiki discussions and training materials that can be archived and recorded. Online instructors are virtually available, respond quickly through email, and generally are prepared to work with diverse student needs. If done well, online nursing programs can enable nurse educators to better facilitate optimal educational experiences for students (Cobb, 2011).

BACKGROUND

Online learning can be seen as a wave of the future that provides access to careeradvancement opportunities for many people—especially for associate degree holders who want to advance their career to a higher degree in a particular field. Although methodologies used to deliver online learning are diverse and well documented in the education and technology literature, ranging from video conferencing, satellite access, and Internet delivery (webinars, Skype, Ovo, learning management systems, and so on), the learning and development experiences derived from designing an online RN to BSN program could be valuable and replicated in many other institutions and developing countries.

As post-secondary education is becoming more accessible than ever and online education is viable for those with busy lifestyles, associate degree nursing (ADN) holders seem to be a ripe target for such technology ventures. This is especially pertinent since some states in the United States are deciding whether to finalize Bills that would mandate all ADN nurses must obtain a baccalaureate degree in nursing (BSN) to continue working in acute care hospitals. According to Hart and Morgan (2010), although online programs are relatively new in nursing education, the number continues to expand due to the demand. However, they also point out that it is important that the planning of any distance learning program starts with the development of effective learning communities. Learning communities offer a social context for learning that greatly enhances the knowledge acquisition of students (Tilley, Boswell, and Cannon, 2006).

Many institutions, particularly in developing countries are finding it very difficult to develop online programs due to a lack of qualified personnel who can train faculty instructors to use new technologies (Rajesh, 2003). Likewise, it is challenging to keep all personnel abreast of forever changing learning technologies. A lack of adequately trained personnel is an impediment to the smooth growth of any online distance learning program.

Costs of system maintenance are included in the planning phase. This is due to the fact that frequent usage may render the system non-functional thus maintenance needs to be continuously supported. As well, sufficiently trained staff, high capacity servers, and system- friendly attitudes, knowledge and skills in the users are all essential for risk reduction during the planning phase (Ranesh, 2003).

Our online program came into being in July 2010 when Howard University, Division of Nursing in Washington, DC decided to integrate the first online RN to BSN degree with the already existing traditional undergraduate program in order to extend the strategic planning of the Health Sciences division. This program was designed to meet the needs of adult students, especially Associate Registered Nurses, who seek baccalaureate study in preparation for career advancement.

At present, the third cohort will be graduating in May 2013 and 100% of the second cohort students initially enrolled in this program have been retained. Program support, technology support, and social support from peers encouraged the RNs to "stay the course" and complete the requirements to graduate (Davidson, Metzger, and Lindgren, 2011). Hopefully, review of this program will contribute to the health sciences goal of identifying best strategic planning practices, so that online programs are sustained in terms of quality, effectiveness, and accountability. As this article reflects, the initial efforts in the program assessment are a starting point but small sample size and developing instruments may restrict accurate interpretation of a concrete summative evaluation in this study.

METHODS

The RN to BSN Track is a program of study for the RN with an associate degree or diplomato study for a BSN Degree. Students are awarded thirty one credit hours from their previous nursing program of study and may complete the degree requirements in a minimum of one year of full-time study or longer for part-time study. The program of study starts in the summer and continues for two full semesters or more for part-time students. Students can complete all courses and graduation requirements through synchronous and asynchronous online distance learning.

The online program was implemented in four phases. The initial phase started with the development and incorporation of informatics into the new curriculum according to the American Association of Colleges of Nursing objectives. This led to phase two which entailed the development of a program brochure and flyers for RN recruitment from the University hospital and ended with student admissions. The third phase was focused on the expansion of online examinations in the entire undergraduate program. The fourth phase focused on the integration of e-documentation which will prepare students to fit into the paperless status that all acute hospitals in the United States must assume in 2014.

Our online program commenced with two consecutive weekend orientations to familiarize the students with the activities of the program. For the first weekend, a mandatory face-to-face workshop was offered to preview the Division of Nursing customized course web page. In these "Orientation Days," advisory sessions were also offered and conducted. The incorporation of recommendations such as introducing a uniform course web page, providing orientation to e-learning systems and promoting the usefulness of the e-learning system have made the online program more user-friendly for the students. Additional information about synchronous and asynchronous learning methods, scholarly writing, APA format, plagiarism, literature search, search engines, and portfolio presentation were also included in the orientation. Technology training is also made available to new students during Orientation Days as well as through the school computer laboratory by our Informatics nurse throughout the semester.

Traditionally, the Division of Nursing used the Blackboard learning management system for student communication and grading but few instructors have incorporated instructional technology beyond the use of e-mail for communication and the Internet for assignment submissions. The launch of this new program included the development of online syllabi organized in distinct modules, course activities and assignments to meet the existing traditional course objectives within an online environment. The Division of Nursing expanded the use of Blackboard add-on capabilities as well to enhance synchronized and a-synchronized teaching methods for the new online program.

A phase-in period of two semesters allowed this development from traditional to partially online with a 100% online program available within six months. The faculty course development was not funded and no workload credit was awarded, thus the process took longer than usual to complete. The program uses multiple technologies such as e-mail, student-produced video to present an assignment, wikis, blogs, and the virtual classroom in Blackboard, as well as Webinars for one of the elective courses.

THE REVIEW: ONLINE SURVEY DESIGN AND ANALYSIS

At the end of the second semester, student qualitative data were collected via a survey with two main sections, focused on:

1. students' satisfaction about the program and perspective about the online faculty and
2. impact of the online program on student professional and personal growth.

As well, an online survey about the students' satisfaction of the online program, students perspective about the online faculty and the impact of the online program on the students professional and personal growth was conducted using a 6 point Likert scale questionnaire {(very low (1), low (2), medium (3), high (4), very high (5), not applicable (0)} to generate quantitative data about the online program.

This quantitative data were analyzed to determine the outcomes of the program using 24 variables as depicted in Tables 15.1 and 15.2. The data were subjected to descriptive, chi-square, and analysis of variance (ANOVA) statistics to analyze these variables and guide model development.

TABLE 15.1 Student Perception and Satisfaction of the Program

VARIABLES	VERY LOW (1)	LOW (2)	MEDIUM (3)	HIGH (4)	VERY HIGH (5)	N/A (0)
Student expectations		1 (14.23%)	3 (42.86%)		4 (57.14%)	
Earned grade worth the expense and time commitment		1 (14.23%)	1 (14.23%)	4 (57.14%)	1 (14.23%)	1 (14.23%)

Instruction in terms of flexibility compared with traditional (classroom) instruction experienced before or since		2 (28.57%)	5 (71.43%)	1 (14.23%)
The overall quality of the faculty		1 (14.23%)	4 (57.14%)	3 (42.86%)
Faculty dedication to quality learning experience		1 (14.23%)	4 (57.14%)	3 (42.86%)
Faculty accessibility		1 (14.23%)	5 (71.43%)	2 (28.57%)
Faculty receptivity to academic concerns	1 (14.23%)	2 (28.57%)	4 (57.14%)	1 (14.23%)
Quality of education compared to other online educational programs you have attended.		1 (14.23%)	6 (85.71%)	1 (14.23%)
Level of satisfaction with the educational experience		2 (28.57%)	4 (57.14%)	2 (28.57%)
Level of satisfaction with the academic performance		1 (14.23%)	5 (71.43%)	2 (28.57%)
Comparison of the education to that of your co-workers and professional peers		1 (14.23%)	4 (57.14%)	3 (42.86%)

Table 2 showed the frequency of the student professional and personal growth responses according to different levels from very low to very high and not applicable as shown below.

TABLE 15.2 **Professional and Personal Growth Responses**

VARIABLES	VERY LOW (1)	LOW (2)	MEDIUM (3)	HIGH (4)	VERY HIGH (5)	N/A (0)

Likelihood of selecting Howard University. Division of Nursing online program again if you were in the process of choosing?		3 (42.86%)	4 (57.14%)	1 (14.23%)
Overall assessment of the program		3 (42.86%)	5 (71.43%)	
Overall satisfaction with the program		2 (28.57%)	6 (85.71%)	
Feeling as part of the Howard University DON family		2 (28.57%)	6 (85.71%)	
Gaining meaningful knowledge from the program		1 (28.57%)	6 (85.71%)	1 (14.23%)
Improving my analytical skills		3 (42.86%)	3 (42.86%)	2 (28.57%)
Opportunities to apply theory to real issues		2 (28.57%)	4 (57.14%)	2 (28.57%)
Innovative teaching	1 (14.23%)	2 (28.57%)	3 (42.86%)	2 (28.57%)
Career preparation/Job enhancement		2 (28.57%)	6 (85.71%)	
Intellectual growth/ stimulation		1 (14.23%)	6 (85.71%)	1 (14.23%)
Personal growth		1 (14.23%)	6 (85.71%)	1 (14.23%)
Social and cultural awareness		1 (14.23%)	5 (71.43%)	2 (28.57%)

FINDINGS

Out of the eight students that were initially enrolled in the program, twenty five percent had previous online learning experience while seventyfive had none. The study shows that the students preferred the flexibility of the online learning compared with the traditional classroom instruction experience. Career preparation/job enhancement was a significant factor when quality of education was compared to other online education the student had (see Table 15.3).

Table 15.3 shows that career preparation and job enhancement were significant, $X^2 (2, N = 8) = 8.000, p = .018$ when the quality of education at Howard was compared with other online education attended.

TABLE 15.3 Quality of education compared to other online educational programs attended versus Career preparation/Job enhancement

	VALUE	DF	ASYMP. SIG. (2 SIDED)
Pearson Chi-Square	8.000[d]	2	.018
Likelihood Ratio	8.997	2	.011
Linear-by-Linear Association	4.971	1	.026
N of Valid Cases	8		

$X^2 (2, N = 8) = 8.000, p = .018$

Faculty dedication and faculty satisfaction were highly significant when compared with overall quality of the program with 99.6% of the predictors explained in this study (see Table 15.4).

Multivariate Analysis

Table 15.4 shows that faculty dedication and accessibility were highly significant, $R^2 = .996$, $F(6, 8) = 75.593, p < .013$, when compared to the overall quality of the program with 99.6% of the predictors explained.

TABLE 15.4 Multivariate Analysis—Linear Regression Model

					CHANGE STATISTICS				
Mode l	R	R^2	Adjusted	SE	R Square Change	F Change	df1	df 2	Sig. F Change
1	.998[a]	.996	.982	.469	.996	75.593	6	2	.013

$R^2 = .996, F (6, 8) = 75.593, p < .013$

Finally, the linear regression model generated from the statistical output showed that overall assessment of the program was predicted by the faculty characteristics, professional/personal gain and level of satisfaction (see Figure 15.1).

Figure 15.1 shows the comparison between instructions of flexibility with the traditional classroom instruction experience.

This model could be used in the future by any institution planning on integrating online teaching/learning tools into their program. This model has shown that faculty characteristics, students' professional/personal gain and satisfaction of the program must be considered prior to implementation of any online learning.

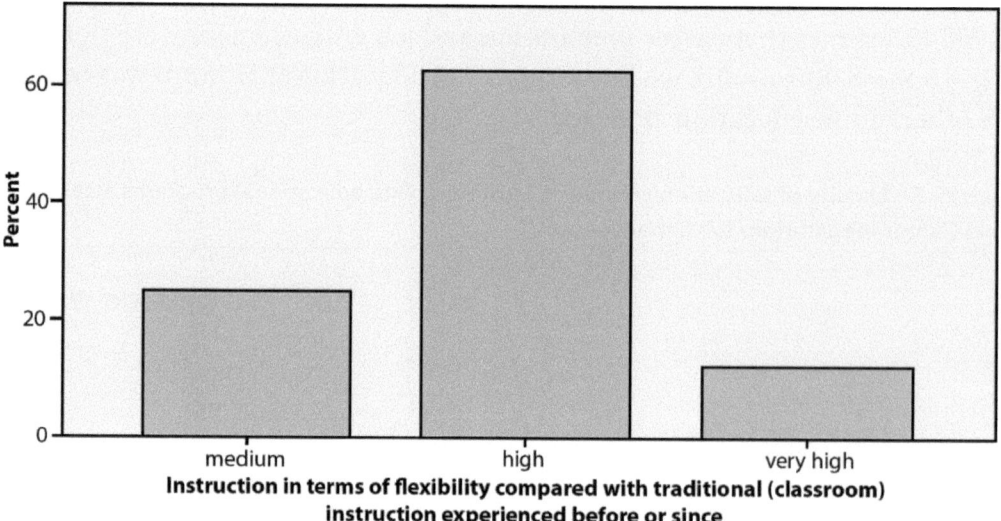

FIGURE 15.1 Instruction in terms of flexibility compared with traditional (classroom) instruction experienced before or since

DISCUSSION AND CONCLUSION

A significant difference was found in perceived professional values depending on level of nursing education, position or title, and professional organization membership. The highest level of perceived professional values was expressed by RN-BSN students when compared to other registered nurses with associate or lower degrees in nursing (Kubsch, Hansen, and Huyser-Eatwell, 2008). RN to BSN students described their pursuit of a BSN as a "journey of being" and "becoming professionals" (Rush, Waldrop, Mitchell, Dyches, 2005).

Our RN to BSN online program is a positive venture to empower registered nurses who may not be able to obtain their BSN due to numerous responsibilities and busy schedules. The choice of system and design of online programs are of paramount importance to ensure that the objectives and goals of the project are met and fulfilled. In the planning phase when considering which system to use, the school should consider acquiring a server that would meet and exceed the capacity of the program activities as it grows, as well as its cost effectiveness, user friendliness and pedagogic value. Results from the present study provide collaborative evidence regarding students' satisfaction related to this particular online program. Most of the students embraced the online program and wanted all of the traditional nursing courses and programs to be offered online.

SIGNIFICANCE OF THIS STUDY

Additional courses using hybrid programs have been developed and implemented in our Nursing Leadership and Informatics and Technology courses. The Graduate Nursing Division has launched a online Nurse Educator track in January 2012 due to the success of this RN-BSN online initiative. Finally, other universities and colleges could replicate the Nursing model for online implementation with good strategic planning that resist impending risks. Similarly, courses could be developed to meet the needs of people living outside the United States.

RECOMMENDATIONS

Overall, there should be consideration for qualified personnel, continuous system maintenance, faculty training, tools needed for delivery, flexible methods, friendly usability, likeability, knowledge and incorporation of adult learning principles and incentives for instructors to develop their online teaching knowledge and skills. Future study would also be enhanced by using more students (higher sample size) for more reliable and validated results.

References

Cobb, S. C. (2011). Social presence, satisfaction, and perceived learning of RN-to-BSN students in Web-based nursing courses. *Nursing Education Perspective. 32*(2):115–9.

Davidson, S. C, Metzger R, & Lindgren, K. (2011). A hybrid classroom-online curriculum format for RN-BSN students: cohort support and curriculum structure improve graduation rates. *Journal of Continuing Education in Nursing, 42*(5):223–32.

Hart, L. & Morgan, L. (2010). Academic integrity in an online registered nurse to baccalaureate in nursing program. *Journal of Continuing Education in Nursing, 41*(11):498–505.

Kubsch, S., Hansen, G., & Huyser-Eatwell, V. (2008). Professional values: the case for RN-BSN completion education. *Journal of Continuing Education in Nursing, 39*(8):375–84.

Rajesh, M. (2003). A Study of the problems associated with ICT adaptability in Developing Countries in the context of Distance Education. *Turkish Online Journal of Distance Education- TOJDE, 4*(2). http://tojde.anadolu.edu.tr/tojde10/articles/Rajesh.htm

Rush, K.L., Waldrop, S., Mitchell, C., & Dyches, C. (2005). The RN-BSN distance education experience: from educational limbo to more than an elusive degree. *Journal of Professional Nursing 21*(5):283–92.

Tilley, D.S., Boswell, C. & Cannon, S. (2006). Developing and establishing online student learning communities. *Computers and Informatics in Nursing, 24* (3):144–9

Technology Integration in Undergraduate Traditional Nursing Programs: Students Online Testing Experience

By Priscilla O. Okunji, Ph.D., RN-BC and Mary H. Hill, DSN., RN,
*Howard University, College of Nursing and Allied Health Sciences,
Washington DC, Division of Nursing*
E-mail Address: priscilla.okunji@howard.edu

ABSTRACT

Introduction: This article describes a pilot study conducted to survey senior nursing students' responses to online testing preference and the efficiency of the Blackboard® system to offer such testing.

Methods: Preparation for online testing was done in phases starting with the planning for the testing space and computer availability. This was followed by selection and uploading of appropriate questions on the course Blackboard® site for student access. The questions were then exported to the testing port of the course web page with certain embedded restrictions. Finally, the survey was developed with seventeen items based on a review of the literature and implemented. Data analysis was performed on student responses on the survey, and results indicated moderate to high support for online testing.

Findings: The survey analysis indicated that more than half of the students preferred online exams over traditional testing, indicating likability and convenience over traditional scantron paper exams. Most students showed a preference for online testing and recommended that test results be available for immediate review. One advantage to introducing online testing was to foster familiarity with computerized testing as preparation for the NCLEX-RN® licensure exam. However, a disadvantage was that the Blackboard® system lacked the capacity for comprehensive statistical analysis for test item discrimination.

Key Words: Online Education, Testing, Learning, Technology, Online Tests, Blackboard®

INTRODUCTION

Many institutes of higher learning are integrating technology and informatics to promote innovation in the process of teaching and learning. Instructors are looking for efficient ways to deliver content and assessment. Advances in educational technologies are increasing at a rapid pace. The technology explosion creates a challenge for nursing faculty to stay current on existing and emerging technological developments. Today's students expect information to be timely and engaging, and resources availed through technology provide opportunities to enhance learning environments (Price, Handley, Millara & O'Donovana, 2010). The numbers of online programs continue to expand (Hart & Morgan, 2010). According to Salamonson and Lantz (2005), more programs in higher education are adopting hybrid formats of course delivery and learning. The hybrid online learning with traditional classroom teaching offer effective and flexible course delivery without the complete loss of face-to-face contact. Online testing (use of information technology for any assessment-related activity) is another opportune application of technology, and readiness for online testing before integrating in nursing courses is an important consideration.

BACKGROUND

The technology explosion of e-learning may have major benefits for nursing education, especially with the current shortage of faculty (Neuman, 2006). Online teaching and learning are being increasingly adopted in both medical and nursing educational programs (Cook et al., (2008); Lewis, Davies, Jenkins & Tait, (2001); Reime, Harris, Aksnes & Mikkelsen, (2008); Tegtmeyer, Ibsen & Goldstein, (2001)). According to Ormrod (2011), course factors of relevance and design influence a learner's decision to persist or drop a course even after enrollment. Nurse educators today face many challenges including how to design imaginative and innovative ways to educate future nurses (Rich & Nugent, 2010). Integration of technology in the classroom is becoming common with many colleges introducing technologies such as smart stations (electronics fitted with a built-in microprocessor); audience response tools (such as Clickers) and smart phones (e.g. Blackberry, iPhone, Android). Web 2.0 (defined as a new version of World Wide Web that allows users to interact and collaborate with each other in a social media dialogue) applications such as blogs, forums, and wikis are also being used as components of Course Management Systems (CMS).

Blackboard® is a popular Web-based server CMS that features convenient course management, customizable open architecture, and scalable design, allowing for integration with student information systems and authentication protocols. Simulations like SimMan (medical simulation mannequins, models or related artifacts) and virtual patients (interactive computer simulations used in healthcare education) are also in use in some nursing schools.

According to Chaffin and Maddux (2004), the evolution of technology has vitally influenced nursing education and is continually gaining greater importance. The Internet enables the students to learn in the classroom, remotely, or at home. Some nurse educators are now adapting traditional content with ease by using alternative teaching methods that integrate Internet technology (Chaffin & Maddux, 2004). Nelson et al, (2006) highlighted potential benefits of vital educational information systems for nurse faculty. The authors reported that although faculty manage large amounts of data, that only a few automated systems have been created to assist faculty to improve teaching and learning via the management of information related to individual students, the curriculum, educational programs, and program evaluation.

Fetter (2009) described how substantial evidence links information technology (IT) with improved patient safety, care quality, access, and efficiency, but cautioned how nurses must demonstrate competencies in computers, informatics, and information literacy in order to use technology effectively for practice, education, and research. The author further reported that the profession has established technology competencies for both beginner and experienced nurses and newly revised standards have been articulated for advanced practice nurses. Unfortunately, there is a critical concern that many nursing students do not have these requirements and that nurse educators are not prepared to remedy this.

The literature suggests that technology competency is still at novice skill levels for most faculty and students. In the USA, deficits in technological competencies are a significant concern, because of the federal government mandate of full implementation of Electronic Health Records (EHR) by 2014. It is a known fact t that EHR will require all nurses to use technology to deliver, document, and obtain reimbursement for patient care. This is the rational for the introduction of SimChart in many undergraduate schools to simulate EHRs before students graduate and join the paperless healthcare work environment.

Creedy et al, (2007) conducted a study to explore graduating Bachelor of Nursing (BN) students' perceptions of a Web-enhanced learning environment, their computer literacy skills, and use of technology, and how these influenced their satisfaction. The results showed a 64% (n = 170) response rate. The authors provided Web-enhanced learning opportunities by integrating online activities and content such as quizzes, videos, and virtual laboratories to augment on-campus and off-campus learning approaches. The authors reported that more than half (61.4%) of the students reported having competent skills, while the quality and usefulness of the Web-enhanced material was rated as fair to above average. However, the students' perceptions of technical and faculty support for Web-enhanced learning was rated low (Creedy et al, 2007). Overall the authors reported that satisfaction with the Web-enhanced program was associated with level of technology skills and perceived quality and usefulness of the online material. The authors reported that statistical analysis of the factors contributing to the students' overall satisfaction of a Web-enhanced learning environment included literacy skills, access, perceived quality, usefulness, and support) and accounted for 18.5% of the variance. The authors concluded that as more nursing programs use Web-based resources, greater attention should be given to the initial assessment and development of students' information literacy skills. As well, students with good technology skills are more likely to perceive Web-enhanced material as useful.

Kock, et al (2010) reported that tailoring information to the needs of the students is an critical strategy in today's modern classroom. The authors described how web-based learning support, informed by multimedia theory, including interactive quizzes, glossaries with audio, short narrated Power Point presentations, animations and digitized video clips were introduced in a first year Bachelor of Nursing biological sciences course at an university in metropolitan Sydney. The authors enrolled all students and invited them to access the site then recorded the number of hits to the site using the student tracking facility available on WebCT (the course management system used in their program). The authors showed that 80% of students enrolled in the subject accessed the learning support site and that the students' perception of the value of the learning support site was assessed using a web-based survey. The survey was completed by 123 participants, representing a response rate of 22%. Three themes emerged from the qualitative survey data concerning nursing students' perception of the web-based activities: 'enhances my learning', 'study at my own pace', and 'about the activities: what I really liked/disliked'. The authors concluded that web-based interventions, supplementing a traditionally presented nursing science course were perceived by students to be beneficial in both learning and language development.

Another study by Rouse (2007) entailed the adoption of a computerized database for testing and analysis to promote and evaluate the nursing student's critical thinking skills and prepare them to write the National Council Licensure Examination (NCLEX) exam after graduation. According to Schmidt & Stewart (2009), faculty members are challenged to create meaningful learning activities that enhance online nursing education. The authors discussed the implementation and usage of Second Life as an innovative Internet-based strategy to engage students in active learning. As well, Campbell and colleagues (2008), concluded that a research methods course could be web-based and found that increased online activity was associated with higher assignment marks. The authors highlighted how new opportunities for educational research have emerged through the use of virtual learning environments such as the Blackboard® system to routinely record the activities of learners and instructors. Many schools with online programs use Web 2.0 applications, such as forums, wikis, blogs, and virtual classrooms to enhance online interaction with students. Other sophisticated social media are being used by some, such as Second Life (an online virtual world that enables users, called Residents, to interact with each other through avatars) to provide real-time (synchronous) interaction.

Online testing is another example of technology integration in nursing education. Some authors argue that information should be tailored to a learner's unique needs for effective and flexible learning (Park & Choi (2009); Koch et al. (2010); Glinkowski & Ciszek, (2007); Mangunkusumo et al. (2007); Ruiz, Mintzer & Leipzig (2006)). Online testing as a method of assessment has not been widely adopted in traditional programs yet due to space, computer availability, technical concerns, security and reliability of the testing system, and student and instructor comfort levels. Instructors have contemplated about whether students should write exams in classrooms due to concerns about space. Yet at the same time instructors worry about the integrity of tests if students write them online without supervision, or need technical assistance.

Authors such as Wu et al., (2006) warn about unsuccessful online learning, but several other studies (Kock, (2010), Salamonson and Lantz, (2005), Bloomfield, Roberts & White, (2010); Cook et al., (2008) and Moule, (2006)) have demonstrated some positive outcomes of e-learning and testing. Online tests offer numerous advantages including access and convenience which encourage student time management skills. Students also instantly see the result of their test because the results are automatically generated to give immediate feedback. Furthermore, after the tests are scored, the data statistics are immediately loaded in the grading folder for instructor access and interpretation. Another major benefit of online testing is the time savings for grading compared to traditional pencil and paper shading and scantron grading (Newman, 2000). Many schools are going digital due to time management, accuracy cost, and access of digitally stored grades.

Traditionally, the Division of Nursing in our institution used the CMS for student communication and grading but few had incorporated instructional technology for research, classroom assignments or quizzes in general. Preparation for online testing was done in phases starting with the planning for the testing space and computer availability. This was followed by selection and uploading of appropriate questions on the course Blackboard® site for student access. The questions were then exported to the testing port of the course web page with certain embedded restrictions. Finally, the survey was developed with seventeen items based on a review of the literature and implemented. Data analysis was performed on student responses on the survey, and results indicated moderate to high support for online testing.

The Division of Nursing expanded the use of the CMS recently by incorporating a new online program, Blackboard® that included synchronized and a-synchronized teaching methods. The University recently adopted this new CMS to met our unique teaching and learning needs. Blackboard® offers custom applications to help one adapt the Blackboard Learn™ platform to meet unique needs and preferences and to and create tailored applications for students and educators.

According to the Blackboard Learn™ plus (2011), custom applications feature CMS building blocks™ development to deliver a custom software solution that was reported to have been professionally designed and tested. This new version of CMS enhances and extends learning to meet course specific requirements. It also includes the necessary information, technical exercises, development examples, and documentation to allow administrators to effectively manage the application. As well, the new integration and customization maintenance tools provide the reliability of ongoing support for the custom application (Blackboard Learn™ plus, 2011). Unfortunately, this CMS platform does not compute test item analysis. This component is necessary because it enables instructors to recognize, focus on and teach content that students are weak on.

Class evaluation can be done online in both traditional and online program but whether the current Blackboard® CMS version is efficient in reflecting test results and student friendly is not clear. This study focused on a pilot experience of recent online testing in an undergraduate traditional nursing course to determine if Blackboard® CMS is an effective tool for online testing.

METHODS

The online testing was implemented in phases. The initial phase started with the planning and securing space in three separate sites: Health Sciences Stokes Library Informatics room with 15 computers, Division of Nursing Learning Resource Center (LRC) with 14 computers and the remaining students (8) were housed in the lecture room (ISAS 100) with their wireless laptops. This led to item analysis and creation of the questions within the institution`s Blackboard® system. The third phase involved exporting the questions for student use after inserting all the control cues including the timing and password for access. The fourth step was the creation of questions for the survey which generated the data for analysis. The survey questions were coded using a likert scale with points of very high (5), high (4), moderate (3), low (2), very low (1) and not applicable (0). Two exams were given and supervised by instructors at the three separate sites for each exam.

PARTICIPANTS AND ETHICAL CONSIDERATIONS

The participants (n = 37) were senior students enrolled in a Nursing Leadership and Management course and the online survey was administered via the Blackboard® CMS (see Table 15.1). The survey submission was anonymous to avoid identification of participants (blind submission). The survey was voluntary and ethical approval from Howard IRB was obtained prior to the submission of this paper.

TABLE 15.5 Baseline Characteristics of Students (n = 37)

VARIABLE	NUMBER	PERCENTAGE
Gender		
Male	5	13.5%
Female	32	86.5%
Age Group		
<24	23	62.6%
25–35	10	27.0%
36–46	4	10.8%
First time Online Testing		
Yes	22	59.0%
No	15	40.5%

DATA ANALYSIS

Data were collected via the online survey, presented in Blackboard® at the end of the 2011 spring semester and quantitatively analyzed for frequency of response to explore student perceptions and satisfaction related to 17 variables. The survey information was tallied and entered into the variable table as shown in Table 15.2.

TABLE 15.6 Student Perception and Satisfaction Levels of the Online Testing

VARIABLE	VERY HIGH	HIGH	MEDIUM	LOW	VERY LOW	NO RESPONSE
Comfort level in computer usage	29.7%	45.9%	21.6%	0%	2.1%	0%
The convenience of taking traditional exam online	13.5%	37.8%	35.1%	13.5%	0%	0% *(Continued)*

TABLE 15.6 Student Perception and Satisfaction Levels of the Online Testing (Continued)

VARIABLE	VERY HIGH	HIGH	MEDIUM	LOW	VERY LOW	NO RESPONSE
The likelihood of taking online exam again	10.8%	35.1%	37.8%	5.4%	10.8%	0%
Advantages of the online exam over traditional scantron paper exam	8.1%	21.6%	54.1%	8.1%	8.1%	0%
Online exam likability over the traditional scantron paper exam	5.4%	27.0%	48.6%	10.8%	8.1%	0%
Preference of the system showing the questions one at a time in a window	10.8%	27.0%	45.4%	5.4%	10.8%	0%
Preference of the system showing all the questions at the same time in a window	10.8%	21.6%	45.9%	13.5%	8.1%	0%
The system allowing students complete all the questions at a set time	5.4%	37.8%	35.1%	16.2%	2.7%	2.7%
The system allowing the students exiting a test and continuing the test from the last question they answered	21.6%	51.3%	24.3%	0%	0%	2.7%
The preference of using an online testing system enables students get used to a similar environment as they would find themselves working in today's paperless acute care	8.1%	37.8%	48.6%	2.7%	0%	2.7%
Growth of online exam is a reality for most colleges	13.5%	56.8%	27.0%	0%	0%	2.7%
Online testing environment is in line with an online "NCLEX" or other proficiency online type exams which is becoming more popular	18.9%	37.8%	29.7%	10.8%	2.7%	0%
Within the exam-taking period, I can break and resume where I stopped	18.9%	45.9%	32.4%	2.7%	0%	0%
I don't have to wait until next class to find out what I made on the exam because I can obtain my score immediately after taking the exam	40.5%	29.7%	24.3%	2.7%	2.7%	0%

All data were subjected to statistical analysis available in the Blackboard® CMS to ensure meaningful results. General data analyses were conducted in the following order. First, descriptive statistics was used to summarize students' demographics, experiences, perspectives and satisfaction level. Next, Excel was used to table the baseline characteristics of the students (Table 15.1) and finally, the students' perception and satisfaction levels of the online testing were represented as shown in Table 15.2.

RESULTS

The findings of the study showed that the majority of the students were female, less than 24 years of age and less than half (40.5%) had never had online testing experience.

BASELINE CHARACTERISTICS

Of the 37 students surveyed, all completed the questionnaires for a response rate of 100%. As shown in Table 15.1, 13.5% were males while the remaining were females (86.5%). Many of these students were young adults with ages ranging from < 24 (62.2%), 25–35 years (27.0%) and 36–46 years old (10.8%). The results also indicated that fifty nine percent of the students had previous online testing while 40.5% had none.

SURVEY FINDINGS

Table 15.2 presents the results of student perception and satisfaction levels of the online testing which indicate that students have **very high** perception and satisfaction on "I don't have to wait until next class to find out what I made on the exam because I can obtain my score immediately after taking the exam,' (40.5%). This was followed by students' **high** perception and satisfaction on, "growth of online exam is a reality for most colleges," (56.8%) "the system allowing the students exiting a test and continuing the test from the last question they answered," (51.3%), "Within the exam-taking period, I can break and resume where I stopped," (45.9%); "being comfortable in computer level" (45.9%) and "Online testing environment is in line with an online "NCLEX" or other proficiency online type exams which is becoming more popular" (37.8%).

The students' **medium/moderate** perception and satisfaction were "advantages of the online exam over traditional scantron paper exam," (54.1%) "online exam likability and convenience over the traditional scantron paper exam," (48.6%), "The preference of using an online testing system enables students to get used to a similar environment as they would find themselves working in today's paperless acute care," (48.6%), "preference of the system showing all the questions at the same time in a window," (45.9) and "preference of the system showing the questions one at a time in a window,"(45.4%).

Qualitative student comments on how the online testing could be improved for more likeability included:

1. "I like the idea of the test still being proctored, as opposed to taking the exam at home, because that is how NCLEX is."
2. "The more practice the better. It is good preparation for NCLEX."
3. "After get use to it maybe it will increase my ability to take on line test."
4. "More practice and online exams at junior level."
5. "Having taken exams online in other classes and an online class in the past, I don't mind online exams."
6. "I think that the time limit and remaining time should be specified at the top of the screen. Also results should be available immediately. I like the idea of showing fewer questions on the screen as well (maybe 10 questions instead of all 50)."
7. "Finding my score out right away after I take it. And doing it on working computers."
8. "As long as we can go back after completing exam to recheck our answers. Taking exam online is not a bad idea; I have to get use to it."
9. "It's okay how it is now."
10. "Given adequate time, and opportunity for a break if needed."
11. "Practice assignments online."
12. "It is an innovative step and prepares us for the real world, which is progressing rapidly from paper based to information technology."
13. "More time to take the exam."
14. "Ability to take a break."
15. "Ability to take the exam at my own time."

DISCUSSION

Key benefits of online testing identified by the students centered on the relevance of online testing to other online tests they must take, including NCLEX and preparation for work environments tests, and being able to see their results immediately after the test. Our results showed promising responses to the online testing, indicating high likeability and positive student perceptions and satisfaction (Chen and Chuang, 2012). These positive effects are in keeping with other reported studies (Kock, (2010), Salamonson & Lantz, (2005), Bloomfield et al., (2010); Cook et al., (2008) and Moule, (2006)).

However, the main concern for future use of the Blackboard® CMS for online testing was its limitations for comprehensive statistical analysis of grades and test item responses. The system's statistical result output only gives basic statistical analysis of frequency, mean, mode, median, and standard deviation with no test item analysis for each question.

As well, students commented that it could be more user-friendly if the CMS settings/controls could be adjusted by the test-taker to present a determined number of questions on the screen (such as all questions, one question, and so on) and if the test-taking could be paused so they could go for break as needed, then resume where they left off without loss of allotted test time.

CONCLUSION

The results indicate that students engaged favourably with the online testing and wanted more in other courses. Based on this result, it could be concluded that the system is well suited for certain tests such as quizzes and other homework assignments that some instructors have already initiated online. However, exams with many questions (50 or more) that require item discrimination for students benefit may need a more robust system. Hopefully, Blackboard® will evolve by redesigning system components that could feature expanded statistically-driven results that are required in today's innovative summative program evaluations.

LIMITATIONS

A limitation of this study is that a small sample of students (n=37) and only the senior students were used. A second limitation was that the survey questions may have been biased and leading. The validity of the study tool could have been increased if the students' perspective and satisfaction survey was delivered by another faculty other than the course instructor and was examined by experts for validation prior to administration.

FUTURE PLANS

We shall continue to use the Blackboard® platform for both online and traditional testing but will continue to search for supportive exam software that would complement Blackboard® and accomplish the goal of our technology integration into the curriculum with needed test item analysis outcomes. Repetition of this pilot study will utilize a larger sample size from different classes and courses and the survey questions would be validated and delivered by a neutral individual to avoid bias.

References

Blackboard Learn plus. (2011). *Custom applications*, Retrieved May 19, 2011 from http://www.blackboard.com/Platforms/Learn/Services/Implementation-Services/Custom-Applications.aspx

Bloomfield, J., Roberts, J. & While, A. (2010). The effect of computer-assisted learning versus conventional teaching methods on the acquisition and retention of handwashing theory and skills in pre-qualification nursing students: a randomized controlled trial. *International Journal of Nursing Studies, 47*(3), 287–294

Campbell M., Gibson W., Hall A., Richards D., Callery P. (2008). Online vs. face-to-face discussion in a Web-based research methods course for postgraduate nursing students: a quasi-experimental study. *International Journal of Nursing Studies, 45*(5):750–9.

Chaffin A. & Maddux C. (2004). Internet teaching methods for use in baccalaureate nursing education. *Computers and Informatics in Nursing, 22*(3):132–42.

Chen, H. Y. & Chuang, C. (2012). The learning effectiveness of nursing students using online testing as an assistant tool: A cluster randomized controlled trial. *Nurse Education Today 32* (3):208–213.

Cook, D. A., Levinson, A. J., Garside, S., Dupras, D. M. Erwin, P. J & Montori, V. M. (2008). Internet-based learning in the health professions: a meta-analysis. *Journal of the American Medical Association, 300* (10), 1181–1196.

Creedy, D. K., Mitchell, M., Seaton-Sykes, P., Cooke, M., Patterson, E., Purcell, C. & Weeks, P. (2007).Evaluating a Web-enhanced bachelor of nursing curriculum: perspectives of third-year students. *Journal of Nursing Education, 46*(10):460–7.

Fetter, M. (2009). Improving information technology competencies: implications for psychiatric mental health nursing, *Issues in Mental Health Nursing, 30*(1):3–13.

Glinkowski, W., Ciszek, B. (2007). WWW-based e-teaching of normal anatomy as an introduction to telemedicine and e-health, *Telemedicine and e-Health 13*(5), 535–544.

Hart, L. & Morgan, L. (2010). Academic integrity in an online registered nurse to baccalaureate in nursing program. *Journal of Continuing Education in Nursing, 41*(11):498–505.

Koch, J., Andrew S, Salamonson Y, Everett B, Davidson P. (2010). Nursing students' perception of a Web-based intervention to support learning. *Nurse Education Today, 30*(6):584–90.

Lewis, M. J., Davies. R. Jenkins, D. Tait, M.I. (2001). A review of evaluative studies of computer-based learning in nursing education. *Nurse Education Today, 21*(1), 26–37.

Mangunkusumo, R. T., Brug, J., Duisterhout, J. S., de Koning, H. J., Raat, H. (2007). Feasibility, acceptability, and quality of Internet-administered adolescent health promotion in a preventive-care setting. *Health Education Research, 22*(1), 1–13.

Moule, P. (2006). E-learning for healthcare students: developing the communities of practice framework. *Journal of Advanced Nursing, 54*(3), 370–380.

Nelson, R., Meyers, L., Rizzolo, M. A., Rutar, P., Proto M. B., Newbold, S. (2006). The evolution of educational information systems and nurse faculty roles. *Nursing Education Perspectives, 27*(5):247–53.

Neuman, L. (2006). Creating new futures in nursing education: Envisioning the evolution of e-nursing education. *Nursing Education Perspectives, 27*(1), 12–15.

Newman, C., 2000. Online testing rated. *Advertising-Age, 71*(20), p 64.

Ormrod, J. E. (2011). Social cognitive views of learning. In Smith, P.A. *Educational psychology: developing learners* (pp.352–354). Boston, MA: Pearson Education, Inc.

Park, J. H., & Choi, H. J. (2009). Factors Influencing Adult Learners' Decision to Drop Out or Persist in Online Learning. *Journal of Educational Technology & Society, 12*(4), 207–217. Retrieved from Academic Search Premier database on May 19, 2011.

Price, M., Handley, K., Millara, J., & O'Donovana, B. (2010). *Assessment & Evaluation in Higher Education, 35* (3), 277–289. DOI:10.1080/02602930903541007

Reime, M. H., Harris, A., Aksnes, J., Mikkelsen. J. (2008). The most successful method in teaching nursing students infection control–E-learning or lecture? *Nurse Educator Today, 28*(7), 798–806.

Rich, K. L., Nugent, K. (2010). A United States perspective on the challenges in nursing education. *Nurse Education Today, 30*(3):228–32.

Rouse, D. P. (2007). Implementation of a computer database testing and analysis program. *Computers and Informatics in Nursing,* 25(5):273–80.

Ruiz, J. G., Mintzer, M. J., Leipzig, R. M. (2006).The impact of e-learning in medical education. *Academic Medicine,* 81(3), 207–212

Salamonson, Y., Lantz, J. (2005). Factors influencing nursing students' preference for a hybrid format delivery in a pathophysiology course. *Nurse Education Today, 25*(1):9–16.

Schmidt B., Stewart, S. (2009). Implementing the virtual reality learning environment: Second Life. *Nurse Educator, 34*(4):152–5.

Tegtmeyer, K., Ibsen, L., Goldstein, B. (2001). Computer-assisted learning in critical care: from ENIAC to HAL. *Critical Care Medicine, 29* (8), N177–N182 suppl.

Wu, J. P., Tsai, R. J., Chen, C. C., Wu, Y. C. (2006). An integrative model to predict the continuance use of electronic learning systems: hints for teaching, *International Journal on E-learning,* 5(2), 287–302.

Printed by Libri Plureos GmbH in Hamburg, Germany